Praise for *Dr. Nita's Crash Course for Women*

"Inspires women to celebrate their womanhood, teaches them to embrace their sexuality, and encourages them to take control of their health. I have no doubt that this witty, informative book will educate and uplift women around the world. It is a must-read!"

— **Andrew Ordon, MD, FACS**, host of *The Doctors*

"Dr. Nita is an incredible doctor, educator, and human being. She works tirelessly at providing scientific information to the public in a pragmatic and digestible way and empowers people to take action and improve their health and wellness. Her empathic, personable, and engaging speaking style is second to none, and people all over the world have been transformed by Dr. Nita's work."

— **Dr. Judy Ho**, clinical and forensic neuropsychologist and author of *Stop Self-Sabotage*

"Highly witty and readable yet comprehensive, Dr. Nita's book allows every vulva owner to take charge of their sexual health and empowers them to ask informed questions about their bodies at their gynecology appointments. I highly recommend keeping *Dr. Nita's Crash Course for Women* on your bookshelf and never using Dr. Google again."

— **Paria Hassouri, MD**, pediatrician and transgender healthcare provider and author of *Found in Transition: A Mother's Evolution during Her Child's Gender Change*

"This is the ultimate guide to women's health, with practical information, poignant stories, and answers to all the questions we may not be brave enough to ask but need the answers to. Thank you, Dr. Nita, for this warm and informative guide to health and living better."

— **Saloni Sharma, MD**, author of *The Pain Solution*

"*Dr. Nita's Crash Course for Women* is a great read. This book invites us to ask important questions of ourselves, while delivering much-needed health and medical information in an accessible way. Oh yeah ... and Dr. Nita is laugh-out-loud funny. Enjoy!"

— **Dr. Rosalyn Dischiavo**, author of *The Deep Yes: The Lost Art of True Receiving* and president of American Association of Sexuality Educators, Counselors and Therapists (AASECT)

"As a woman of color, a wellness practitioner, and someone who has struggled with severe hormonal disruption (large fibroids, endometriosis, dysmenorrhea), I appreciate the expert perspective from another woman of color. Each chapter of *Dr. Nita's Crash Course for Women* has great takeaways that are easy to understand and implement. But most importantly, the reader will feel empowered with the tools they need to navigate their health journey."

— **Jovanka Ciares**, herbalist, wellness expert, and author of *Reclaiming Wellness*

"I will highly recommend this book! As an ER doctor, and as a husband who just watched his wife go through all the ups and downs of pregnancy and labor, I know how important access to trusted information is for women who have questions about their bodies as they go through life. Dr. Nita is the perfect resource to help women better understand their 'womanhood,' and she has done a great job in this book of being a friendly yet professional resource for anyone who has questions that maybe they've been too afraid to ask."

— **Travis Stork, MD**, *New York Times* bestselling author of *The Lose Your Belly Diet*

"I love what Dr. Nita is about. I love her stance and her commitment to fostering healthy dialogues between women and their doctors. The world needs to have these types of conversations."

— **Lisa Nichols**, *New York Times* bestselling author of *Abundance Now* and motivational speaker

"A must-read for every woman. Dr. Nita connects the dots between a vibrant sex life and optimal health."

— **Mike Dow, PhD, PsyD**, *New York Times* bestselling author of *The Sugar Brain Fix*

DR. NITA'S

CRASH COURSE
FOR WOMEN

Better Sex, Better Health,
Better You

DR. NITA'S

CRASH COURSE
FOR WOMEN

NITA LANDRY

MD, FACOG, OB-GYN   COHOST OF *THE DOCTORS*

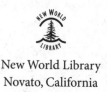

New World Library
Novato, California

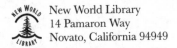

New World Library
14 Pamaron Way
Novato, California 94949

Illustrations © Bigstock.com: pages 275 and 276. Illustrations © Medicalimages .com: pages 17, 19, 28, and 225. Illustrations © Shutterstock.com: pages 23, 25, 189, 190, 192, 264, 288, 302, 344, 346, 349.

Text design by Tona Pearce Myers

Library of Congress Cataloging-in-Publication Data

Names: Landry, Nita, author.
Title: Dr. Nita's crash course for women : better sex, better health, better you / Nita Landry, MD, FACOG, OB-GYN, Cohost of *The Doctors*.
Description: Novato, California : New World Library, [2022] | Includes bibliographical references and index. | Summary: "A medical doctor and respected cohost of CBS's Emmy Award-winning show *The Doctors* offers an edgy and fun guide to women's health"-- Provided by publisher.
Identifiers: LCCN 2022029688 (print) | LCCN 2022029689 (ebook) | ISBN 9781608687541 (paperback) | ISBN 9781608687558 (epub)
Subjects: LCSH: Women--Health and hygiene--Popular works. | Gynecology--Popular works.
Classification: LCC RA778 .L36 2022 (print) | LCC RA778 (ebook) | DDC 613/.04244--dc23/eng/20220722
LC record available at https://lccn.loc.gov/2022029688
LC ebook record available at https://lccn.loc.gov/2022029689

First printing, October 2022
ISBN 978-1-60868-754-1
Ebook ISBN 978-1-60868-755-8
Printed in Canada

New World Library is proud to be a Gold Certified Environmentally Responsible Publisher. Publisher certification awarded by Green Press Initiative.

10 9 8 7 6 5 4 3 2 1

For my mom and dad

Contents

Part II. Common Women's Health Issues: Advocate for Your Health Like a Pro

Illustrations

Figures

Tables

My Story

How I Got This Way and What It Can Do for You

When I was a little girl, I wanted to be a doctor *and* what I called a "TV interviewer person." So I spent a disturbingly large portion of my childhood reading science encyclopedias and chasing my sisters around the house as I forced them to participate in fake media interviews (they were not willing participants, to say the least). And I can remember how excited I was in middle school and high school as I told people about my plan to become a doctor and work in the entertainment industry. Just about all of them felt like the doctor part would happen for me. However, some questioned, doubted, and even laughed out loud at my entertainment goals. Because of those negative reactions (along with the low self-esteem that came along with my acne, braces, and overall teenage awkwardness), I quickly learned just how much external doubt can feed self-doubt. And I got a firsthand lesson on how self-doubt could kill my dreams if I wasn't careful. So I stopped discussing my entertainment aspirations. But I never lost sight of them. Even my closest friends and family had no clue, but I had come up with a plan and I was moving in silence. First I would focus on my medical degree. Then I would transition into entertainment — *somehow*.

After high school I kept my entertainment goals tucked away like a dirty little secret for more than a decade as I obtained my biology degree, went to medical school, and completed a medical residency in obstetrics and gynecology (ob-gyn).

At the end of my medical residency, the other residents were applying for "regular jobs," but I knew that wasn't the best choice for me. While I was excited about being an ob-gyn, I also needed to make ample room for my secret dream. Not knowing about my entertainment aspirations, my faculty adviser gave me the perfect solution. He said, "You should think about becoming a traveling doctor." Traveling doctors are hired to fulfill a specific need for a specific period of time when a medical group is short-staffed for some reason. For example, a doctor's office might need someone to fill in if one of their practitioners has to go on medical leave.

This career path would give me the schedule flexibility I needed. Plus, it had the added bonus of allowing me to travel across the country and work with different patient populations. So I decided to go for it. I sold my condo fully furnished and drove into my future, keeping only the things that could fit into my gray four-door sedan that I'd affectionately named Bullet. And just like that, I was officially a traveling doctor.

Over the next several years, I spent time taking care of women from different backgrounds in New York, California, Arizona, Minnesota, Texas, Alaska, and a lot of other places in between. Sometimes I was in a major city, and sometimes I was in the middle of nowhere. And when I say the middle of nowhere, I mean the middle of *nowhere*. On one assignment, the housing options were so limited that I was asked if I was willing to live at an animal shelter that had dogs, cats, baby goats, chickens, and just about every other type of farm animal you can think of running around. Anyone who knows me knows that my answer was a resounding no, but you can ask me more about that if we ever meet in person.

As I traveled across the country, having open and honest conversations with thousands of women from different races, cultures, and socioeconomic statuses, one thing became crystal clear to me: many of us aren't enjoying and embracing womanhood. We are tolerating it. The scariest part? We don't even realize how much healthier and happier we could be. I met thirty- and forty-year-old women who were peeing in their pants whenever they coughed, laughed, or sneezed. They somehow thought that having a "mommy bladder" was just an inevitable, unfortunate consequence of motherhood. (Spoiler alert: I don't care how old you are, it's not.) I met women who could barely function for three to seven days every month because their period cramps felt like a baby elephant was wearing high heels and tap-dancing on their uterus. I met women tolerating mediocre sex. And enduring domestic abuse. And feeling alone and scared during infertility and miscarriage struggles. The list goes on and on and on. If you can think of a women's health issue, I probably encountered it.

But on my quest to help these women, they also helped me. For example, when I was working on a Native American reservation in New Mexico, a lot of my patients had poorly controlled diabetes with dangerously high blood glucose levels. In the midst of counseling them about simple things they could do to have a healthier lifestyle, I started thinking more about my family history and the crappy genes that put me at a higher risk for things like high blood pressure, diabetes, and high cholesterol. Ultimately, during those conversations that were intended to improve my patients' health, I also motivated myself to improve my diet and exercise regimen. And as I spoke to women who were embarrassed or afraid to admit that they were sick and tired of bringing their partner to orgasmic bliss while their partner brought them to... boredom, it made me think more about my conservative upbringing.

Although our struggles were not always exactly the same, those reflective, aha moments made me feel more connected to my patients all across the country. We were growing into and with our womanhood together. These women were more than just patients to me. We were all part of a community with a special bond. It was a sisterhood. And I was loving every minute of it. But then, this happened...

After several years of being a traveling doctor, I found myself working in Wisconsin one winter. I really liked the patients there, but that Wisconsin winter was kicking my butt, to put it mildly. One morning when I was getting dressed for work, I heard the local weatherman say, "It's colder here than it is in the North Pole." As he went on to give more fun facts about the temperature, I came to the realization that my Louisiana-bred body simply was not designed for that type of extreme, wet cold. That weather report was my cue. It was time to take what I'd learned as a traveling doctor and merge medicine and entertainment. In California. Where sunshine existed. So that day, I put in my thirty-day notice at work and bought a plane ticket to Los Angeles.

When I arrived in California, my training in entertainment consisted of what I'd learned while doing plays and being a teen reporter for the news in my fabulous (but small) hometown of Alexandria, Louisiana. So basically I knew nothing. That was very different from the experience of the people I met who had dedicated years to media training. I vividly remember speaking to someone who asked me if I had a reel. I typically ask questions if I don't know about something, but the way they said it made it clear that anyone interested in entertainment should know what a reel was. I replied, "No, I don't have a reel, but I'm working on it!" The truth is, I didn't even know how to correctly spell the word. After I figured out that it was a short promotional video that showcased a person's on-camera skills, I got to work by signing up for a hosting workshop, some acting lessons, and an improv class.

After a few months of training, I picked up a microphone and went out on the streets of Hollywood, where I started asking people random questions like:

- "How many holes do women have 'down there' all together?" (A lot of people don't know the answer to that question. It's three, by the way — the urethra, the vagina, and the anus.)
- "How long is the average penis?" (Hint: Most people expect guys to be walking tripods … they are not.)
- and "What types of cancers can birth control pills help to prevent?" (A couple of them are ovarian cancer and endometrial cancer.)

Using the footage from those interviews and my entertainment classes, I put together a reel, and I put it on my newly created website for the world to see. Then I waited to see if someone (anyone) would like it.

Since I had no connections, no agent, no manager, and practically no television experience, I thought I'd be waiting a long time. But I guess God had other plans, because a few weeks later I opened my email and found that my reel had gotten me an invitation to be a guest expert on a segment of the Emmy Award–winning talk show *The Doctors*. Once I was on set for the taping of the show, I was surprised how *right* it all felt and quickly realized that my limited on-camera training was not going to hold me back — the show was, after all, a medical series, and when it came to discussing the field of medicine, I was right at home. The producers must have felt the same because that guest expert appearance led to becoming a recurring cohost — meaning I got to take part in the entire show instead of just one segment. I guess you could say that first appearance worked out because I became a recurring cohost and worked with the show for the next six seasons.

Since then I've appeared as a medical expert on television programs such as the *Today* show, *Good Morning America, Dr. Phil, Iyanla: Fix My Life, Entertainment Tonight,* and *CBS National News*; I've interacted with viewers from around the world; and I've traveled across the country, speaking at events and colleges. So, as it turns out, my "TV interviewer" ambitions became the best-kept secret I ever shared.

That's my story.

Now I've combined all my experiences to write a book that is filled with practical advice that has the power to help vulva owners around the world evolve into a healthier, happier version of themselves.

A Word about Terminology and Privacy

Terminology

In this book I use the word *woman* and the pronouns *she* and *her* to describe individuals whose assigned sex at birth was female, and I use the word *man* and the pronouns *he* and *him* to describe individuals whose assigned sex at birth was male. However, anatomy does not dictate identity. Therefore, I recognize that people who were assigned female or male at birth may identify as female, male, or nonbinary.

Privacy

As a physician (and as a friend), I talk to people in confidence, and I would never betray their trust. Therefore, the stories in this book do not reflect specific real-life events. Instead, each scenario described combines my personal experiences, as well as the experiences of my family, friends, and the thousands of patients I have had the honor of caring for over the years. All names and identifying information have been changed to protect everyone's privacy. (Exception: The individuals who were kind enough to be interviewed for the transgender chapter specified that they wanted to use their real names.)

Part I

SEX

Let's Have "The Talk"

Chapter 1

Somebody Lied about Sex

Misconceptions about Sex

I had no clue how many lies about sex women believe until I found myself at a "porn party" one night. (Sorry, Momma — yes, I willingly went to one. But let me tell you how it all started.)

Before that night, you never would've caught me at that type of party because I would get hella uncomfortable when anyone talked about sex. I'm talking about an armpit-sweating, zero-eye-contact, fear-of-burning-in-hell-for-eternity kind of uncomfortable. But then when I was in medical school, one phone call from my friend "Joan," an aspiring sexologist, changed everything.

I was at home minding my own business when Joan called to invite me to her house for what she called "an intellectual debate exploring the complexities of porn." When I asked, "What does that even mean?" she described a small gathering for a group of her female friends. There would be wine and cheese, followed by article reviews to discuss the pros, cons, misrepresentations, and social ramifications of porn. Then we would end the night with a viewing party that closely examined the subject matter.

At that point, I thought, "Is she asking me what I think she is? Because it sounds like she's using a bunch of fancy words to ask me to go to her house to eat some cheese, drink some wine, and watch porn videos." Well, as it turns out, that's exactly what she was asking.

Since Joan knew I had very conservative views about sex at that time, she wasn't surprised when I told her I was going to have to pass on her invitation. But Joan doesn't take no for an answer. So she proceeded to explain that I would be missing out on an "anthropological experiment designed to facilitate an intellectually stimulating conversation regarding the billion-dollar porn industry's negative impact on the sexual experiences of women."

At first I laughed and rolled my eyes. *There she goes with those academic words again.* But then I thought about my patients and realized she might be on to something. As a medical student, part of my learning experience was to shadow different doctors. I would watch in awe as they performed groundbreaking surgeries, swoop in with a lifesaving diagnosis, or explain extremely complex medical conditions in easily understandable terms. They were brilliant...*right up until a female patient complained about her sex life.* Then a lot of them were...let's just say, the opposite of brilliant. To be fair, I didn't expect every specialist to address sexual complaints. A general surgeon shouldn't be a patient's go-to person for complaints about low sexual desire. But I was amazed that some of the internists and family-practice doctors — and even a few of the ob-gyns — seemed visibly uncomfortable when a woman wanted to talk about her sex life. Their answer to just about every sexual complaint, big and small, was a vaginal lubricant, vaginal estrogen, or my personal favorite: simply flipping over to try a new sexual position.

And in some cases, women didn't even get offered one of those solutions. Once, while I was shadowing an ob-gyn during my training, a patient told him she had a low sex drive. The doctor smirked as he looked her dead in the eyes and said, "So do most of the other women I saw this morning. Get in line, lady." Then he walked out of the room.

I want to stay professional, so I won't tell you what I thought about his rude, condescending comment, but feel free to let your imagination run wild. What I thought was probably worse.

But I had to admit, despite his very inappropriate response, he wasn't exactly wrong. Woman after woman after woman complained about her sex life that morning. And, sadly, they were all sent away with zero solutions — so there literally could have been a line of women, all desperate to get some sort of real advice on how to resuscitate their sex life.

As I thought about those experiences during my conversation with Joan, common sense told me that pornography wasn't responsible for 100 percent of the sexual dilemmas consuming women. But I also knew Joan was right when she said it was partially to blame. So as an aspiring ob-gyn who wanted to help women who were suffering from what I call "orgasmic deprivation," I decided that her porn party might be a great chance to get some clarity. Maybe hearing more real-world conversations would help me understand why so many patients were struggling with their sex life.

When I arrived that Friday night, the atmosphere at Joan's house felt like a typical book club meeting. At first everyone was professional and chose their words carefully. But as we got more comfortable and emptied a "few" wine bottles, the proverbial cardigans and pearls came off. Then the discussion shifted from "Here is what the study in the article showed" to "Let me tell you what happened to me this one time." Once the viewing party started, everybody's verbal filter was pretty much nonexistent, and small conversations broke out all around the room. As I moved from conversation to conversation, one thing became really clear really fast: as women, we believe a lot of lies when it comes to sex.

The Top Three Lies Women Believe about Sex

I didn't know it that night, but the most common lies I heard at the party would turn out to be the same ones that continue to pop up the most when I talk to my patients. Here are three of the top lies that I hear and what I've learned about those lies over the years.

Note: The people at this gathering were cisgender (meaning their gender identity corresponded with the sex they were assigned at birth), heterosexual women, so the views were limited. But I've learned that these lies are also experienced by people with various gender identities and sexual orientations.

Lie 1: Your partner isn't enjoying your body.

Whether it was because of her thighs, abs, butt, the shape of her vulva, or some other reason, I heard woman after woman admitting she was convinced her partner didn't find her sexy. A lot of the women even avoided sexual positions they enjoyed because they didn't like the way their body looked from certain angles.

What I've learned

While you are being unfairly critical of your body, it's very likely that at the *exact same moment*, your significant other is having a magnificent time enjoying the same body that you are stressing out about. This is especially true when it comes to heterosexual women. How do I know? Research! A recent study from the *Archives of Sexual Behavior* looked at more than

52,500 adults in the United States, including gay, lesbian, bi-sexual, and heterosexual men and women. They discovered that even though we're the ones with the more sensitive plea-sure center (shout-out to the clitoris), men are winning on the orgasmic front. Ninety-five percent of heterosexual men said they usually or always orgasmed when sexually intimate, and the numbers for gay and bisexual men were just a little lower. For women, lesbians had the highest number, with 86 percent of them saying they usually had an orgasm. Bisexual women went down to 66 percent, and heterosexual women came in *last place*, with the least number of orgasms at 65 percent.[1]

Of course, insecurities aren't the only reason heterosexual women are 30 percent less likely to have orgasms than hetero-sexual men, and we'll talk about those other reasons later. But it really bothers me that at this very moment women all around the world are in the middle of sex with a partner who is moan-ing and groaning and enjoying the experience, and instead of doing the same, these women are using their brainpower and energy to conduct a personal body analysis or judge their sex-ual performance.

Sigh. Please stop. Don't let your insecurities get in the way of your orgasm because if you are a heterosexual woman (for example), there's a 95 percent chance that your love handles, thighs, C-section scar, and all the other *perceived* flaws you're unnecessarily fixated on aren't getting in the way of his. You're not perfect, that's true. But nobody is. Including your part-ner(s). So relax the nitpicking about your body and enjoy the ride — pun intended.

Lie 2: If you are a woman, faking orgasms is a part of life. You should accept that fact and move on.

At one point during our porn party, Joan shouted, "Excuse me! Let me hear you clap if you're a sexually active person who has never faked an orgasm." At that point, the room remained totally quiet. Well, except for the voice of the woman in the porn video who apparently didn't have any cash for the pepperoni and pineapple pizza she ordered and had something else to offer. But I digress. The point is that every woman in the room who had ever had sex was guilty of faking it. *But why?*

What I've learned

Many women fake orgasms for the same reasons. Here are three of the most common ones:

1. They don't want to hurt their partner's feelings. This can happen in any relationship, but I see it a lot with patients who have been with their partner for a while. They come to the clinic and tell me, "I have a low sex drive." But for a lot of them, the main problem is a version of, "The sex we have is not the type of sex I want. I love my partner, but I enjoy having sex with them about as much as I enjoy standing in line at the social security office."

2. They're looking for a way to end the festivities because they'd rather be doing something else. Some of these women have unresolved relationship issues that make it almost impossible for them to enjoy sex with their partner. And others are too stressed, overwhelmed, or tired to care that they haven't experienced sexual pleasure in weeks or months — I know that all the mommas who are thinking about things like laundry or buying peanut butter in the middle of sex can relate to this!

3. They're afraid they'll get dumped or cheated on if they don't appear to enjoy the type of sex their partner wants to have. So when they want to start sex with a bubble bath, a soothing massage, and smooth R&B

but he's into whips, chains, bondage, and anal (or vice versa), she goes with what he wants. Because her main goal is his sexual satisfaction, she follows his lead — even if he's leading her down a path with no sexual pleasure in sight. Then, when he has his happy ending, she fakes hers because she's afraid that if she doesn't pretend to enjoy his sexual skill set, he'll go out and find someone who does.

But what are the ramifications of faking it over, and over, and over in a long-term relationship? It may seem convenient or even considerate to lie, but many women who are serial fakers eventually become bored and/or resentful. That's not fair to the woman. And if she's in a relationship with someone who actually wants to please her, it's also not fair to her partner, who was never given a chance to learn what she desires sexually because she or he truly believed that the fake orgasms were real.

I'm not saying you should roll over, gaze into your partner's eyes, and say, "Wow, that sex was really bad." But instead of repeatedly faking orgasms, try to effectively communicate what would make sex great for you. If that's difficult for you, one tip from Dr. Rachel Needle, codirector of the Modern Sex Therapy Institutes, is to take it back to the basics. When you and your partner are just hanging out and doing nonsexual stuff, ask them what they like sexually. That opens the door for a meaningful conversation that focuses on their needs. Hopefully, they'll decide to ask you the same question, but if not, after discussing their needs for a while, you can strategically use the "compliment sandwich technique" to let them know what you like. For example, say, "I love it when you (give them a compliment about something they do sexually); I think it would be great/fun if we (insert what you'd like to do differently); it feels good when you (insert another compliment)."

This conversation might be the first step toward making changes that both of you will enjoy. But in some situations, if your partner isn't willing to have a conversation about what will please you sexually, there might be an underlying issue that needs to be addressed, perhaps in therapy (if you're in a committed relationship).

Lie 3: "Respectable women" should feel shame or guilt if they like porn, stripper poles, or anything else considered inappropriate by societal standards.

One of my favorite observations at Joan's was the interaction between two women who we will call Alexandra and Madison. Alexandra, a middle-aged married mother of three who apparently gets the giggles when she drinks, said that she'd never watched porn because of cultural beliefs. But as I watched her smile and clap as she slowly turned her head to the side to ensure that she was watching the *Mothers I'd Like to ... "Do Stuff with"* (aka *MILF*) video from an optimal angle, it was obvious that she was thoroughly enjoying her introduction to adult videos. She was really rooting for those moms! And Madison, a happily single and sexually adventurous schoolteacher who kept yelling, "I've done that," was the perfect person to guide her through her first porn experience.

Alexandra and Madison were from very different worlds, but they served as a reminder that some women really enjoy porn (and stripper poles and other stuff).

What I've learned

I understand and respect the fact that when it comes to pornography, it's a solid yes or no for some women. But as someone who used to be a strong "hell no," I also understand how it can be a bit of an internal struggle for some people. They're curious about it, but their inner conservative voice tells them it's too provocative and their inner feminist voice tells them that even female-centered "ethical porn" is exploitative and degrading. Plus, in some cases, they can hear their mom's or grandma's voice telling them it's flat-out disgusting.

My opinion now that I've seen women across the country struggling to embrace and understand their sexuality? We need to take the sexual limitations off consenting adults. Grown women should be encouraged to unapologetically like what they like. Furthermore, the world needs to stop acting like a woman can't like literary books, stripper poles, porn, and PTA meetings simultaneously.

So whether you decide that you're a no-porn, no-lights, missionary-style kinda person or you find yourself enjoying flashing lights and fetish porn as you utilize the gynecology stirrups (the things you put your feet in during a Pap smear) that you purchased for your personal use at home, rest assured that there's at least one doctor on this planet who supports your decision wholeheartedly.

Note: If you do decide to watch porn, please do some research on the platform, production company, and performers you are watching to ensure that they don't have complaints against them for unsafe working conditions. And remember that porn is entertainment, not education.

Porn-Party Inspiration

In an unsurprising turn of events, by the end of the night I'd learned absolutely, positively nothing from the videos of the plumber, the pizza guy, or the musician and his muse. But the real-life stories I heard ignited my curiosity.

The number of women who were unhappy with their sex

life that night was way too high. Even higher than I initially thought it would be. And I knew that there had to be a logical reason that so many of them seemed to feel like the odds of having a great sex life were about as high as the odds of them finding a leprechaun sitting on a pot of gold at the end of a rainbow...eating cheese. So as a budding, inspired future physician, I set off with my newfound intel determined to crack the case of lost libidos, painful sex, orgasmic deprivation, "malfunctioning G-spots" (as one woman put it), and all the other pressing issues I heard about that night.

That's what this part of the book is about. I want to tell you about some of the most powerful lessons I've learned since that fateful night when a porn party changed my life. (Ha! I never thought I'd string those words together to make a sentence, but it's true.)

Chapter 2

A Clitoris as Long as a Penis, the G-Spot Debate, and More

Anatomy

A friend of mine had a girlfriend who refused to stimulate his penis during sex. Based on the sex she'd had in the past, she was convinced that she could make him orgasm solely by massaging his perineum (the landing strip of skin between his scrotum and anus). She seemed so sure of herself that he initially went along with her plan, but after several failed attempts, he finally told her that perineal stimulation just didn't do it for him. However, he was sure that he'd cross the orgasmic finish line with a little penile attention. But she refused to listen. She was sure that his previous lovers just didn't find the right angle, pressure, or rhythm. For the next few weeks, she remained laser focused on giving him a perineal-based orgasm. But no matter how hard or long she tried, and no matter how much he wanted her to succeed, his sexual satisfaction was nowhere to be found. Finally, one night she caved in and stimulated his penis, and he absolutely loved it. Just like he knew he would. But despite that undeniable confirmation, she convinced him that they should go back to perineal stimulation. So she went back to her old ways, and his pleasureless nights returned.

I'm lying! No penis owner has ever told me that they were

13

expected to endure a ridiculous situation like that. Why? Sexually speaking, we have realistic expectations when it comes to what works for penis owners. Yes, a lot of women know that some men orgasm when their prostate is stimulated during a perineal massage, so there's nothing wrong with giving perineal stimulation a shot. But we aren't obsessed with making guys orgasm with perineal stimulation. Instead, we understand and respect the fact that the male penis is a very common and logical go-to source for sexual pleasure. So since it would be sexually inefficient (and inconsiderate) to go around intentionally ignoring people's penises during sex, it's not the norm to do that. We know better because we've been taught better.

But when it comes to female sexual pleasure, logical expectations go out the window.

Case in point: the female equivalent of the penis isn't the vagina. It's the clitoris. And just as men enjoy their penises, women enjoy the hell out of their clitorises — so much so that most women who masturbate stimulate their clitoris with little or no vaginal penetration, even when they are using a vibrator.[1] But when those same clitoris-loving females add a penis-possessing beau to the scenario, a lot of them spend the whole sex session focusing on penis-in-vagina (P-in-V) sex — even though in most P-in-V positions it's like the male's penis is in Texas while the visible part of their beloved clitoris is in Minnesota getting absolutely no stimulation. Then, when 75 percent of those women don't orgasm from that vaginal penetration, instead of saying, "Our bad. Vaginal penetration works great for a guy's penis, but we need to switch it up for the ladies," society makes it seem like those women have anatomically inferior vaginas.

But they don't. Malfunctioning female anatomy isn't the problem. A lack of understanding of how female anatomy is designed to work is the problem.

That's why one of the first steps toward fulfilling my porn party–inspired career goal to make this world a better place for female sexuality is to help women understand their anatomy — not in a "this is what happens when an egg meets a sperm" way that will prepare them for an eighth-grade sex ed test but in a way that allows them to confidently call BS when society tells them that their body should be functioning in a way it wasn't designed to function. And in a way that will leave them with the knowledge and confidence they need to politely redirect sexual partners who seem to be a little "lost" during sex.

Wait, What Can That Part Do?

I hear people say that a lot of guys don't know where the clitoris is. And they're right. In fact, I'd bet good money that at this very moment there are well-intentioned grown men on every continent (including Antarctica) who are on the verge of dislocating their jaw as they unknowingly lap away about an inch below their partner's clit. Poor fellas. *However*, don't assume that penis owners are the only ones who don't know their way around down there. Once when I was shooting a social media video, I walked around Hollywood with a diagram of a female vulva and asked more than 150 women to point out the main parts. More than 35 percent of women between the ages of twenty-one and fifty-five couldn't properly identify the clitoris. Most of the vulva owners who got it wrong thought that the clitoral hood was the clit, but the hood is basically the female equivalent of the male foreskin on an uncircumcised penis. And even if they did know exactly where the clitoris was, most females admitted that they had never systematically explored their genitalia to make sure they're taking advantage of all their erogenous zones. (An erogenous zone is a sensitive area on the body that causes sexual arousal when it's touched.)

But in defense of every grown vulva owner who isn't maximizing the potential of their genital region, our society hasn't exactly been a big supporter when it comes to encouraging women to celebrate or explore their sexual preferences. So let's start at the top and work our way down for a crash course that is designed to help you determine what *you* like sexually.

Vulva is an umbrella term that describes the part of the female genitals that you can see when you take off your clothes. Here are the main parts, which are also shown in figure 1:

- Mons pubis
- Labia majora (larger outer lips)
- Labia minora (smaller inner lips)
- Clitoral hood
- Glans clitoris
- Urethra (the tube that releases urine from the bladder)
- Vestibule
- Hymen
- Perineum (pronounced per-IN-ee-um)
- Anus (although we are including it here, technically the anus is a part of the gastrointestinal tract)

Diagrams aren't a great substitution for the real thing. I recommend that you wash your hands and then sit down on a comfortable surface or stand with one foot propped up on a chair or bed. Use a handheld mirror and some good lighting to get some hands-on experience. If the thought of doing this makes you cringe, I want you to ask yourself why. For many vulva owners, the reason is that a part of their subconscious still believes what society teaches us as little girls: that *vulva* and *vagina* are dirty words and dirty things that we shouldn't explore. If that's the case for you, do you still truly believe that, or are you ready and willing to revamp your thinking in the name of sexual pleasure (and liberation)?

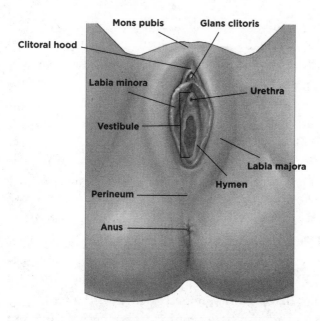

Figure 1. The vulva

DR. NITA'S NOTE
Call It What It Is

Vagina versus *vulva*: Most people call the whole kit and caboodle between a woman's legs her vagina. But the distinction between the vagina and vulva is comparable to the distinction between your mouth and your lips. Like the mouth, the vagina is located inside the body, and like the lips on your face, the vulva is located outside the body. In other words, the vagina is not a part of the vulva, and the vulva is not a part of the vagina.

The mons pubis (aka "mons veneris" or "the mons") is a layer of fatty tissue that sits over the pubic bone at the top of your pubic hairline and extends down to the clitoral hood. Not to go all adolescent memory lane on you, but do you remember the term *dry humping*? Well, thanks to its nerve endings, plus the fact that it's directly connected to the clitoral hood and vulvar lips (translation: when the mons moves, you can get some clitoral movement too), the mons is one of the reasons dry humping was and continues to be such a huge hit in early sexual encounters around the world.

And when it comes to adults who are understandably looking for something more advanced than a good dry hump, a lot of sex experts consider the mons to be one of the most underrated erogenous zones on an adult woman's body. So instead of assuming that it has nothing to offer sexually, spend some time sexperimenting to determine if you've been missing out on some mons-related sexual pleasure. For example, sit one vibrator on your clitoris. And at the same time, place another vibrator on the middle, lower portion of your mons (just above the clitoral hood). Just give it a shot. Your mons might show you a surprisingly good time.

If you move a little farther down, you'll run into fat-filled folds of hair-bearing skin called the labia majora (larger outer lips). Their real claim to fame is protection of your goodies, such as keeping unwanted dirt out of your vagina. But some women also enjoy sexual stimulation of the labia majora.

The two smaller folds of skin found inside the labia majora that don't contain fat or hair are the labia minora (smaller inner lips). In addition to helping the labia majora out with protection, they have supersensitive nerve endings that become even more sensitive when you're sexually stimulated, especially on the inner sides or the edges.

At the top, each of your inner lips divides into two folds that surround the visible part of your clitoris. The fold that's underneath the glans is the frenulum of the clitoris. The flap of skin at the top that arches over the glans clitoris is called the clitoral hood (aka "the hood" or "prepuce," pronounced PRE-pyoos).

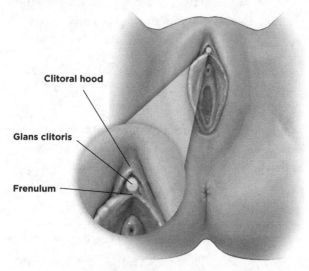

Figure 2. The clitoral hood, glans clitoris, and frenulum of the clitoris

DR. NITA'S NOTE
Tips about Your Lips

As men age, saggy balls are a fact of life, but when is the last time you heard someone talking about scrotal rejuvenation surgery? Probably never, because even though a lot of older men are walking around with balls hanging to their knees, mainstream society doesn't bombard them with unfair judgments.

But when it comes to how aging vulvas look, the world is quick to have a negative opinion. Well, here's my two cents when it comes to what you need to know before you proceed with labiaplasty, which is surgery to change the shape or size of the labia.

The labia majora (outer lips) are usually between seven to twelve centimeters long, but they can be longer or shorter than that. And they come in a rainbow of shades. That means yours could be twice as long and several shades lighter or darker than someone else's but still be perfectly normal and beautiful. Like the labia majora, labia minora also come in a variety of colors, shapes, and sizes.

Some healthcare practitioners diagnose a patient with "labia minora hypertrophy" if their labium (that's singular for labia) measures more than six centimeters when it's stretched from where it attaches to the vulva to its free edge. But not everyone buys into that definition. In other words, there's not a globally accepted definition when it comes to what a "normal" labial shape or size is. So even if your inner lip is wider than six centimeters, most healthcare practitioners (including me) consider it to be within the normal range. Also, remember that your own two lips are probably not going to be identical to each other. As long as they don't itch or burn and you don't have discoloration, lesions, or any other unusual symptoms that need to be evaluated, trust me when I say that your lady lips are healthy and normal.

If you want to make your labia smaller because their size interferes with your menstrual hygiene, disrupts sex, causes discomfort, or simply because of your personal preferences, I support your decision — just make sure you understand the risks and benefits of the surgery, and make sure your surgeon is qualified.

But if you want labiaplasty because unrealistic standards set by society have convinced you that your vulva needs to be "cuter," I encourage you to reconsider. And if you are doing it to please a partner, in my humble opinion, if someone wants to walk out of your life because of the way your labia or some other part of your vulva looks, you should help them gather their things, open the door for them, and wave goodbye as they walk away. You deserve better.

Oh, and to be clear, I actually appreciate the fact that the world doesn't judge a male's worth by how loose his scrotal sac is. All I'm asking is that they keep that same positive energy when it comes to female genitalia.

That's the Spot...Right There!

As far as we know, sexual pleasure is the sole purpose of the clitoris. The average female clitoris, which is made up of several parts, is approximately nine centimeters long. For reference, that's about the length of an average soft penis.[2] The part you see when you look at your vulva (and the only part they usually mention in most textbooks) is the *glans clitoris* — the small nub that's beneath your clitoral hood (shown in figure 2). Let's talk about that part first.

Glans clitoris

The glans clitoris is usually about the size of a pea, but some clitorises are a little smaller or a little larger. This part of the clit is innervated by thousands and thousands of nerve endings. (Just in case you're wondering, that's a lot of nerves!) Approximately 75 percent of vulva owners need this portion of the clitoris to be stimulated in order to reach an orgasm, so as you twist, turn, and flip into different positions, keep that in mind.

DR. NITA'S NOTE
Getting Up Close and Personal with Your Glans Clitoris

If you are really invested in your sexual pleasure, take a mirror and look at how much (or little) of your clitoris naturally peeks from under your clitoral hood without you pulling the hood back. Then, if you can't already see it, gently retract your clitoral hood to look at your glans clitoris. Next, use your favorite lube and the stimulation method of your choice (vibrator, penis, or finger) to get aroused. Once you feel extremely aroused, but before you have an orgasm, look at your clitoris again. It will probably be easier to see because the glans clitoris typically fills up with blood and becomes bigger when a woman is aroused (like a penis, but to a lesser extent, of course). And as this happens, the clitoral hood retracts, making your clitoris more visible/accessible.

Having this information will help you understand your sexual preferences. For instance, if you feel like you need heavy-duty machinery to have an orgasm, it might be because you prefer direct clit stimulation but less of your clitoris is exposed when you are aroused due to a large clitoral hood. In that case, you'd just need to make sure you and/or your partner keep that in mind as you explore ways to ensure that you have adequate stimulation. If needed, you can also gently pull the clitoral hood back during sex.

Take your time sexperimenting to determine whether you prefer direct glans stimulation or stimulation of your clitoral hood. Some vulva owners don't like direct glans stimulation because their clit is very sensitive; others only like it at certain times during sex. Additionally, try out different methods of stimulation. For example, if you are using a vibrator, try different speeds, rhythms, pressures, and angles.

The parts of the clitoris you can't see

Most people think that the clitoris begins and ends with the glans. But when you look at it in its complete, three-dimensional glory, you can see these other parts (figure 3):[3]

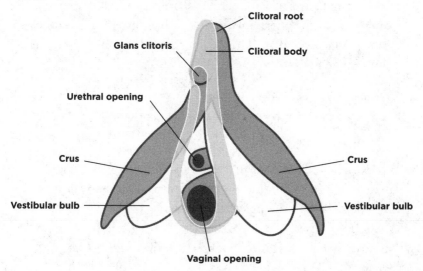

Figure 3. Anatomy of the clitoris

- The clitoral body is two to four centimeters long and connected to the pubic bone.
- On each side is a *crus* (leg), which together in the plural are called the *crura*. They're approximately five to nine centimeters long. They're behind the labia majora (more or less), and they extend deep into the tissue of the vulva.
- The clitoral root connects the clitoral body to the crura. It's just beneath the skin above the urethra, so it's sensitive to stimulation.
- There are also two *vestibular bulbs* (also known as clitoral bulbs), one on each side of the urethra and vaginal openings. These are three to seven centimeters long.

The parts of your clitoris you cannot see are (to put it in extremely simplified, unscientific terms) draped around your urethra, vagina, and labia — sort of like curtains.

Now, the next question is: Sexually speaking, what can these hidden parts of your clitoris do for you when it comes to penetration? The short answer is, maybe a lot, maybe a little, or maybe nothing at all. The long version of the answer can be found in the next section.

The G-Spot Debate and Vaginal Pleasure

In the 1950s a German doctor named Ernst Gräfenberg wrote a paper about a very sensitive orgasm-producing area approximately two inches inside on the front wall of the vagina — the side closest to the belly button (see figure 4). Then in the 1980s, a group of sex experts decided to write a book about this area. Well, when their book, which they called *The G Spot*, became popular, hopeful vagina owners excitedly set out to see what all the fuss was about. And that's where the saga begins. Some women were all smiles after their successful vaginal exploration. But the women who weren't as successful (read: no orgasm) started asking very logical questions, like, "Where the hell is mine?," "Is my G-spot broken?," and "Seriously, is this thing even real?"

Unfortunately, thanks to the lack of research funding for female sexuality, we still don't have all the answers when it comes to the G-spot. But here are what I believe are the top theories explaining why some women have orgasms when this area is stimulated.

Theory 1: Your "G-spot" is actually just your clitoris. Based on this theory, the fate of your ability to have an orgasm from vaginal penetration was decided before you left your mother's womb. Here's why: when you were a fetus, there were hormones floating around to help you develop. Some of those hormones were called androgens. According to some research, the amount of androgen exposure you had determined how far away your clitoris would be from your urethra. The higher the androgen level, the greater the distance. The lower the androgen level, the shorter the distance.

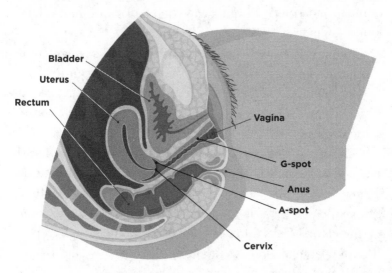

Figure 4. The G-spot and A-spot

If your lower androgen level resulted in your clitoris being less than 2.5 centimeters from your urethra, you are more likely to have an orgasm from penetration. For reference, 2.5 centimeters is around the distance from the tip of the thumb to the first knuckle.[4] (The researchers measured the distance from the clitoris to the urethra instead of the distance from the clitoris to the vagina because they thought it would be easier. And they assumed the distance from a woman's urethra to her vagina was pretty consistent. That assumption is likely not correct, but you get the point of their estimation.)

We aren't sure whether these women have orgasms during penetration because the shorter distance increases the chance that the penis will stimulate the internal aspect of their clitoris or if a shorter clitoral urethral distance increases the chance that the penis will come in contact with their glans during thrusting.

But before you start looking for your tape measure, I want to point out that the researchers measured the study participants using specific techniques. Therefore, an at-home DIY measurement may not be very accurate.

Theory 2: Your G-spot is your urethral sponge. Your urethral sponge is sensitive tissue that surrounds your urethra. When a penis (or something else) bumps against this area as it's thrusting in and out of the vagina, it feels really good to some people.

Theory 3: The truth is a hybrid between theory 1 and theory 2. From woman to woman, the clitoris and urethral sponge vary in size, shape, and location. Maybe the urethral sponge plays a big role for some women, maybe the location of the clitoris plays a big role for other women, and/or perhaps the women who get the most pleasure from the G-spot are those who have anatomy that allows both to be stimulated.

The point is, your G-spot (which actually should be called the G-area since it's not an exact location) has not been proven to be a distinct anatomical structure. Instead, it may just be where your urethra, the hidden portion of your clitoris, and your vagina meet up. And whether or not you experience orgasms when that area is stimulated doesn't necessarily depend on your sexual skill set, your partner's sexual skill set, or your appetite for sex. Instead, it depends on your anatomy. Of course, there's nothing wrong with exploring the possibilities when it comes to vaginal penetration (including other areas like the anterior fornix erogenous zone, "A-spot," which is between the cervix and the front vaginal wall), but I just don't want women who don't orgasm with vaginal penetration to feel like something is wrong with them. And I don't want them to get so fixated on P-in-V sex that it curbs their creativity when it comes to exploring other possibilities for experiencing sexual pleasure.

For example, one study found that 95 percent of women had erogenous zones other than their genitals, and 12 percent of the study participants could orgasm when those spots were stimulated.[5] So instead of being laser focused on penetration, you might be better served doing a Google search for "erogenous zones" and then sexperimenting to find out if your earlobes, the soft spot behind your knees, your inner wrist, or some other part of your body is an orgasmic gold mine.

Ejaculation, Coital Incontinence, and Squirting

About an inch below your glans clitoris, you'll find the opening of the urethra, the three-to-four-centimeter tube that releases urine from the bladder. Under the skin on each side of the urethra, there's a pea-size gland called the Skene's gland (see figure 5). When people talk about ejaculation, squirting (gushing), and coital incontinence, the urethra and the Skene's glands are major players.

Leading experts agree that female ejaculation is a legitimate phenomenon. With ejaculation, a very small amount (one to three milliliters) of a thick, milky white or gray fluid is released from the Skene's glands. This fluid does not shoot out.[6]

Coital incontinence is when you accidentally pee during sex. Experts don't question the validity of that process either.

But when it comes to squirting, which is when a thin, clear fluid comes out of the urethra, not everyone agrees. Some experts believe squirting is actually coital incontinence.[7] Or they say these women are extremely wet and they're simply expelling normal vaginal discharge from the vagina. But other reputable experts argue that squirting is absolutely, positively real.

They say that the fluid from squirting does in fact come out of the urethra — which is the same hole that urine comes out of. But although fluid from squirting may mix with urine that happens to be hanging out in the bladder, the squirted fluid is distinctly different from urine. So these experts believe that fluid from squirting and pee are two different things. But these experts also point out that squirting is not a sign of a superior orgasm. Therefore, there is no need to "chase the squirt." If you squirt, great. If you don't squirt, great. If you are an intermittent squirter...that's great too.

Hopefully, we will continue to have more research on this topic. In the meantime, just have fun.

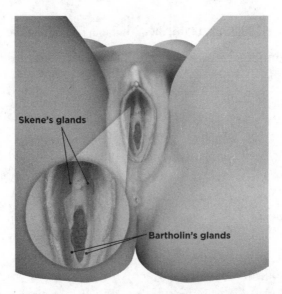

Figure 5. Skene's glands and Bartholin's glands

Some Other Anatomy Stuff You Should Know

- **The perineum.** This is the small hairless area of skin between the bottom part of the labia and the anus. It's full of sensitive nerve endings, with tons of opportunities for pleasure. For those who are into it, caressing or massaging the perineum can result in a lot of pleasure for some people. If you're going to give it a try, just remember to use lubrication and to be gentle.

- **The vestibule.** This is where the vagina and vulva meet. The vestibule skin looks similar to what you find in the vagina, and it's covered by a thin membrane called the hymen, which looks a bit like a ruffled border. From an evolutionary standpoint, we have theories but still don't know why the hymen exists. What we *do* know, however, is that you can tear your hymen doing everything from playing outside or cheerleading to riding a horse. Some vagina owners aren't even born with a hymen. So the myth that an intact hymen proves that a woman is a virgin is just plain junk science.

- **Bartholin's glands.** Bartholin's glands are located on each side of the vaginal opening at the 4 o'clock and 8 o'clock positions. These glands secrete a small amount of fluid to help lubricate the vagina.

Take Ownership of Your Sexual Pleasure

Most women are so busy being disappointed that their body doesn't function in a way that it wasn't designed to function (read: no orgasm during penetration) that they never take the time to lean into and celebrate what their body *can* do. These women, who never systematically explore their body, are unknowingly settling for a sex life that pales in comparison to what they deserve. Don't limit yourself to vaginal penetration. Get curious. Explore the possibilities.

We focused on the genital region, but once you understand the fundamental information that is explained in this chapter, be creative. Think of your exploration as a treasure hunt. Imagine that you have erogenous zones tucked away in nooks and crannies all over your body, just waiting to be discovered.

Don't forget to tell your partner(s) what you learn. Happy hunting ... and stay hydrated.

Chapter 3

(Re)Defining Normal Sex

Desire, Arousal, and Orgasms

Once upon a time, a woman we will call Stacy wanted good sex, but instead she got...John. Here's her story.

In the middle of what was supposed to be foreplay, thirty-five-year-old sexually experienced John started to vigorously rub Stacy's clitoris like he was an intoxicated DJ who was spinning records at a nightclub. Stacy was confused and genuinely concerned about the possibility of getting friction burns on her clit. But when John, who was panting and sweating from all his hard work, noticed that her vagina had produced quite a bit of lubrication, he confidently said, "You're so wet. You like that, don't you?" Then he licked his lips and bit his bottom lip the way that a lot of guys do when they're confident that they're hittin' it right.

Now at this point, Stacy had a decision to make. She could (a) go for the jugular by saying something like, "Absolutely not. This sex is catastrophic"; (b) take control of the situation in a gentler way by saying, "Touch me like this," as she showed him what she liked (this option gets my vote); or (c) protect his ego at all costs by saying, "Yes!"

Welp, Stacy, who really liked John, chose option (c), then she had a fake orgasm shortly thereafter. That decision caused a very proud John to make a mental note of his success, and that DJ trick became one of his signature moves that haunted Stacy and her clitoris for the rest of their relationship.

I'll go out on a limb and say that this exact scenario has probably never happened to you — gosh, I hope it hasn't — but stories like this are exactly why this chapter is needed. While this example focuses just on vaginal lubrication, for every John who doesn't understand that vaginal lubrication doesn't mean a woman actually likes what's happening, there are dozens of other people (of all genders and sexual orientations) who don't understand some other common need-to-know facts about what should be considered normal when it comes to the female sexual experience. And there are way too many women like Stacy, willing to sacrifice their sexual pleasure.

So in this chapter, we'll focus on some problematic misconceptions that unnecessarily wreak havoc on the female sexual experience. Specifically, we'll (re)define what should be considered normal when it comes to three major components of the female sexual response cycle: desire, arousal, and orgasms. If you are interested in learning more about the topics in this chapter or the next, I highly recommend Dr. Emily Nagoski's book, *Come as You Are: The Surprising New Science That Will Transform Your Sex Life*.

Understanding and Embracing Your Sexual Desire (aka Libido) Style

"Low libido" is the most common sexual complaint that women express. But a lot of women who think they have a low or nonexistent libido actually just have a libido that is terribly misunderstood. Here's why.

As it turns out, there are two ways people experience sexual desire. One way is known as spontaneous desire. This is the sexual desire style that most women think they're supposed to have. With spontaneous desire, it's like your sexual desire is right below the surface. So almost anything can get you all hot and bothered. For instance, you may be walking into the grocery store to buy some orange juice, and your purse strap brushes up against your nipple. That simple nipple tap ignites your sexual desire. And now you're thinking, "You know what would go great with my orange juice? Sex!" Or when your partner asks, "Want to have sex?" it's an immediate, "Yep!" for you. Within thirty seconds, your shoes are off, your shirt is halfway unbuttoned, and your brain is prepped and primed to knock some pictures off the wall (or if you prefer a bit less athleticism, you're ready to make passionate love).

Another way to experience sexual desire is called *responsive desire*. This is the sexual desire style that most women actually have.[1]

Unlike spontaneous desire, it takes more effort to find your responsive desire since it's not as close to the surface. You have to put in some effort to get to it. Here's an example of how responsive desire might show up. Sandra and Gina are watching television on the couch during a date night. Gina leans over and kisses Sandra. Technically, sexually neutral Sandra isn't craving an orgasm when Gina kisses her, but she wants to be close to Gina for nonsexual rewards like emotional intimacy, bonding, commitment, affection, and acceptance. So because she is craving those nonsexual benefits, sexually neutral Sandra leans into Gina's kiss. Then one thing leads to another, and Sandra starts to feel physically aroused. Once that arousal reaches a certain threshold, Sandra thinks, "I know I started off just wanting an emotional connection, but this feels really, really good." Then, just like that, sexually neutral Sandra has managed to get her responsive desire ignited, and she gets some nooky.

Note: Of course, consent is nonnegotiable. That means Sandra is a willing participant every step of the way. There's no coercion, and there are no expectations. With responsive desire, you are saying, "Let's get started and see where this goes." Sometimes it might lead to sex, and other times you might just end up enjoying the pleasures of first base. You have the right to end the festivities at any time.

So what are some of the problematic misconceptions? First of all, most women have never heard of responsive desire. They think that spontaneous desire is the only type of sexual desire that exists. So they believe they should walk around craving sex for pretty much no reason. And when they don't find themselves daydreaming about sex while they wash clothes, sit in business meetings, or … watch paint dry, they think something is wrong with them. For a lot of my "honey, not tonight" patients who schedule an appointment with me to talk about their "low libido," learning about responsive desire is an aha moment that changes their life. Once they understand that

spontaneous desire → willingness to be aroused →
the "ta-da" of sexual pleasure

AND

willingness to be aroused → *responsive desire* →
the "ta-da" of sexual pleasure

are both perfectly acceptable ways to get to ta-da, they are relieved. After a brief chat, these women who walked into my office thinking they were broken walk out understanding that the way they experience sexual desire is 100 percent normal.

But I'll admit that some women give me the side-eye when I go into my "embrace your responsive desire" spiel. Not because they don't believe it exists, but because they feel like responsive desire is a second-place prize.

Well, if you happen to be reluctant to accept your responsive desire sexual style, I have three things for you to consider. First of all, the only reason most of you think you should have spontaneous desire is that you were taught it's the only "normal" way to experience desire. But that thinking is outdated. Second, research shows that within the first few years of a relationship, it's very common for a female's predominant desire style to switch from spontaneous to responsive. So even if you started off as a carefree "let's tear each other's clothes off all the time" spontaneous desire person, as you build a life together (read: work, kids, aging parents... drama with your in-laws), it's common to evolve into a "let's bond and figure out how to deal with life" responsive desire person. And last but not least, research shows that spontaneous desire doesn't lead to better orgasms than responsive desire. That has to count for something!

DR. NITA'S NOTE
Some People Don't Desire Sex, and That's 100 Percent OK!

Approximately 1 percent of the population is asexual. According to the Asexual Visibility and Education Network, an asexual person is someone who does not experience sexual attraction. This isn't a definitive guide, but if you think you might be asexual, try answering these questions:

- Is your sexual attraction to others nonexistent or very rare?
- Do you want to have sex or participate in sexual practices?
- If you want to date or get married at some point, would you like sex to be a part of the relationship?
- If you've had sex or engaged in sexual practices before, did you like the experience? Do you want to have sex again?

Asexuality, which isn't the same as abstinence or celibacy, means different things to different people. Some people are asexual all their lives, and some aren't. Some asexual people masturbate, some don't. Some have sex with a romantic partner solely for the emotional connection, and some don't have sex at all. There isn't a right or wrong way to be asexual.

Perhaps you're not satisfied with the spontaneous desire or responsive desire that you experience, or you and your partner are struggling with mismatched libidos. We'll address those issues in the next chapter. But the takeaway from this section is that whether you always experience spontaneous desire, you always experience responsive desire, or you find yourself enjoying a mixture of both, you are healthy and normal. So repeat after me: "Responsive desire isn't low libido. Responsive desire isn't low libido. Responsive desire *is not* low libido!"

Now that we've talked about sexual desire, let's talk about the arousal that might come before or after it.

The Scoop on Sexual Arousal

I think that male misconceptions about vaginal lubrication are one of the biggest problems that heterosexual women don't know they have. Let's talk about how female arousal works and why your partner needs to understand this concept if you want great sex.

The reason a woman who has 0 percent interest in sex can have a vagina that's like a miniature replica of Niagara Falls and a woman who genuinely wants sex can have a vagina that's extremely dry is due to a phenomenon called arousal nonconcordance. With arousal nonconcordance, your level of genital arousal doesn't correlate with how aroused you feel mentally — that's my professional way of saying that either your vagina is wet but you don't feel horny or your vagina is dry when you do desire sex.

The best description of arousal nonconcordance I've seen comes from sex educator Dr. Emily Nagoski. Here's my interpretation of how she explains it: The first step toward vaginal lubrication is seeing, hearing, smelling, tasting, touching/feeling, or imagining something you consider sexually relevant because your mind has been programmed to link that situation to sex. Notice that *liking* what you see, hear, smell, taste, touch/feel, or imagine is not required. That's because when it comes to sexual relevance, liking doesn't matter. The only thing that matters is if your past experiences taught you to associate that situation with sex. Your list of what counts as a "sexually relevant" scenario will be different from your next-door neighbor's. However, as an example, watching a porn video or having someone touch their vulva is sexually relevant to most people.

Whenever you see, hear, smell, taste, touch/feel, or imagine something that you've been conditioned to deem sexually relevant — like "John the DJ" DJing your clitoris — your vagina doesn't care how much your brain actually likes that sexually relevant stimulus at that particular moment. Instead, your vagina makes a unilateral decision and agrees to participate in an automatic, involuntary process that increases its blood flow. And that increased blood flow to the vagina is what ultimately leads to your increased vaginal lubrication.[2]

At the same time that your genital region is ramping up its blood flow, your brain is independently scanning your environment and your subconscious/conscious to decide whether you actually like the sexual stimulus that you are seeing, hearing, smelling, tasting, touching/feeling, or imagining. If your brain decides that you don't like or enjoy the sexually relevant thing that led to your vaginal lubrication, or it's just not a good time for you to have sex for some reason, your brain says, "Nope! I'm not aroused." And you are left with genital arousal but no mental arousal, like Stacy.

And, to be 100 percent clear, contrary to popular belief, arousal nonconcordance has nothing to do with hidden messages, secret fantasies, or "shy" women who are too embarrassed to say what turns them on during sex. In research that looked at a woman's vaginal arousal and brain activity at the same time, it was confirmed that genital response and brain activity frequently don't overlap. In fact, when you break the numbers down, there's only a 10 percent overlap between how aroused a woman's genitals are and how aroused her mind is.[3]

Plus, in addition to vaginal lubrication that happens as a result of increased blood flow to the genitals, cells of the vagina and cervix make vaginal discharge. And it's normal for the amount and consistency of vaginal discharge to change throughout the month based on hormone levels. So if you're at a point in your menstrual cycle when your body is producing more discharge, your partner could mistake that slippery feeling for arousal.

Long story short, the phrase *You're so wet* has been given way too much power. Wetness is not body language for sexual desire or enjoyment. Just like a guy can have an erection without being mentally aroused, women can have increased vaginal lubrication without being mentally aroused.

DR. NITA'S NOTE
When Being Misinformed Gets Dangerous

(Trigger warning: This text box contains information about sexual assault/rape.)

Not understanding why females have vaginal lubrication can actually be dangerous in some situations. While they are being abused, some sexual assault/rape survivors will experience vaginal lubrication. Needless to say, the fact that they experience lubrication definitely doesn't mean they desire the encounter, and it doesn't mean that the abuse is being enjoyed. The lubrication occurs because penetration is sexually relevant. Vaginal lubrication is not consent. And vaginal lubrication should never be used to determine how much someone is enjoying something sexually. Period.

Now let's flip the script. What about vaginal dryness? If blood flow to the vagina is an automatic, involuntary process, why is it that a woman can have a vagina that feels as dry as the Sahara Desert when she sees, hears, smells, tastes, touches/feels, or imagines something sexually relevant and she is actually enjoying that sexually relevant thing or situation?

I mentioned that the increase in vaginal blood flow is what ultimately leads to vaginal lubrication. Well, anything that decreases blood flow to other parts of the body can also decrease blood flow to the vagina. That decreased flow means that you have less blood to work with to get your lubrication going. Here are some reasons that might happen:

- Smoking
- Diabetes
- High blood pressure
- Atherosclerosis (plaques of fatty material in the arteries)
- A low estrogen level for any reason[4]
  - Reasons for a reversible decrease in estrogen include, but are not limited to, being postpartum, breastfeeding, or using hormonal contraception.
  - Reasons for a permanent decrease in estrogen include, but are not limited to, menopause, perimenopause (the transitional period leading to menopause), or surgical removal of the ovaries.

Of course, vaginal lubrication isn't pure blood, it's fluid that is filtered from the blood. Once the blood shows up, lots of factors determine how much fluid will be filtered. For instance, some women naturally produce less lubrication than others because their vaginal walls are less permeable, meaning it's harder for the fluid to pass through, due to genetic factors.[5] It's just the way their vagina functions. And that's totally OK. Lower levels of estrogen come into play here too since decreased estrogen also leads to less permeable vaginal walls.

Some other reasons for vaginal dryness include:

- Over-the-counter cold or allergy medication that is designed to dry out your mucous membranes — because, unfortunately, the meds don't just work on your respiratory tract
- Thyroid disease
- Vaginal infections
- Some antidepressants
- Vaginal douching

The overall health of the vaginal tissue that is being lubricated also comes into play. Additionally, another more practical issue to keep in mind is that the process of getting the blood flowing down there and using that blood flow to create vaginal lubrication takes time. And some people need a lot more time than others. So if you're a slower lubricator and your partner is trying to have wham-bam-thank-you-ma'am sex, your vagina might not be ready . . . yet. If you have more time, slow down and enjoy the process. If you are looking for a quickie instead of a marathon, no worries. A little lube can make you wet on demand. And if low estrogen is your issue, you might benefit from a vaginal moisturizer or vaginal estrogen. For tips on vagina-friendly lube selection or for information about vaginal moisturizers and vaginal estrogen, see pages 334–36.

Note: The Bartholin's glands and the Skene's glands that we discussed in chapter 2 help out with vaginal lubrication, but most of a woman's lubrication comes through the walls of the vagina.

Orgasms versus Sexual Pleasure

Last but not least, let's talk about orgasms and sexual pleasure. One of the reasons women like Stacy feel compelled to fake orgasms is because we're taught that having an orgasm is like giving someone a standing ovation after sex, while not having one is like booing them. In other words, we're taught that (aside from reproducing) climaxing should be the goal of sex. But leading sex experts are encouraging people to change that mentality. Instead of focusing on orgasms, sex experts want people to focus on sexual pleasure. Here's one of the best analogies I've heard sex experts use to explain why the world needs to ditch its obsession with orgasms.

Great sex is like a five-star dining experience. It starts when the bread is brought to the table, and it ends when you grab a peppermint as you walk out the door. Your orgasm, which is like the dessert, is a nice part of the meal. But pleasure comes from the whole meal, from start to finish. And just like it's possible to have a great meal without dessert, it's absolutely, positively, with 100 percent certainty possible to have incredible sex without having an orgasm.

Sex experts want people to remember that sexual encounters are about all the moments. The glance across the table in the middle of dinner that says, "Meet me in the bathroom. I wanna show you something." The giggles that follow you awkwardly getting your arms stuck in your shirt. Or when you're just holding each other and enjoying the nonorgasmic benefits of sex like emotional closeness, bonding, commitment, affection, love, and acceptance.

When you put all the emphasis on having an orgasm, you deprioritize all the other pleasurable moments that a lot of women value as much as (and sometimes even more than) orgasms. Plus, when orgasms are considered a mandatory *requirement* for "successful sex" instead of a pleasurable *option*, both people are focused on "crossing the finish line."[6] That extra stress will actually decrease the probability that you'll orgasm.

Another common misconception is that if it does happen, an orgasm is supposed to feel a certain way. For example, in the last chapter, we learned that the clitoris has a visible portion called the glans clitoris and parts that you can't see, which are draped around the urethra, vagina, and vulva, kinda like curtains. We also learned that there are other vaginal spots that *some* women enjoy having stimulated. Well, it turns out that orgasms that happen when these various areas are stimulated can feel very different because the nerves that travel between each of these areas and the brain are different.

In one study, participants described orgasms from stimulation of the glans as a localized, intense feeling that was physically satisfying, and they described stimulation of the deep areas of the vagina/cervix as a full-body experience that was stronger and longer than orgasms from glans stimulation. But even though the orgasms felt different, according to the participants, there was no clear subjective winner between the two descriptions.[7]

And, of course, your mindset and what's happening in your life are going to impact how your orgasm feels. So even if you strike the same nerves two nights in a row, it's perfectly normal for the feel of an orgasm to vary from sexual experience to sexual experience in the same woman. Sometimes an orgasm might make you feel a sense of peace, like you're floating on air. Other times it might seem like fireworks are exploding in your body (in a pleasant, nonfatal kind of way). And other times it's somewhere between those two extremes. All these ways are normal.

I once saw a woman wearing a T-shirt that said "Orgasms are like chocolate. Some might be better than others, but they're all pretty great." I agree.

Congratulations, You're Normal!

To sum things up, just about everything that most sexually active adults believe about the female sexual response cycle is inaccurate. But we can change that. Even if we have to do it one conversation at a time. So let's start a movement.

The next time you are out with your girlfriends, bring up the topic of responsive desire because it's very likely that one of them needs to know about the concept.

The next time you are speaking to a friend who has sex

with vagina owners, ask them if they know that a female's vagina is not a reliable spokesperson when it comes to her mental arousal.

And the next time you are at a dinner party and you need a topic for small talk as you introduce yourself to people, try, "Hi, I'm (insert your name). What do you think about the current push to have people start focusing more on sexual pleasure and less on orgasms?" Just kidding. (Unless you're willing to do it.) #JoinTheMovement

Chapter 4

Something Isn't Right with My Sex Life. Fix It!

Diagnosing and Treating Sexual Dysfunction

"Katrina" loved her husband, but she just didn't want to have sex anymore. She wanted to want it. She wanted to want him. But no matter how hard she tried, she just didn't. At all. She spent thousands of dollars on countless sex toys and contraptions. She pretended to be everyone from a naughty student, nurse, and police officer to Wonder Woman and a professional wrestler. She even pretended to be from the magical land of Wakanda. She lit candles. He sent flowers. In a moment of desperation, she even bought a book that guaranteed it would improve her sex life, and they embarked on the book's "eighteen ways to ride" challenge. While she was impressed with her flexibility and overall skill set, even her spectacular riding skills didn't get her aroused enough to ignite her responsive desire. So night after night after night ended exactly the same way: with minimal sexual pleasure for Katrina.

Like other people with sexual dysfunction, Katrina wanted her body to want sex as much as her heart did. But nothing she did seemed to help.

She is not alone. In the United States, approximately

40 percent of women have some concerns about their sex life, and 12 percent of those women are distressed about their sexual problem(s).[1] This chapter is for all the women who can see a little bit of themselves in Katrina.

Sexual Dysfunction Quizzes

First of all, I want to point out that most people have sex lives with ebbs and flows. For instance, if you are a new mom who can't figure out how many days ago that Fruit Loop you just found ended up in your hair, it's normal for you to have a "No thanks, I'm good" attitude when it comes to sex. And it's also perfectly normal for ebbs and flows to happen "just because." However, if you've been in a sex slump for months and/or the sex slump bothers you, you can take action.

Here are some quizzes you can take to see if you might have sexual dysfunction, which is defined as difficulties in libido (sexual desire), arousal, orgasm, or pain with sex that are bothersome to the person experiencing the symptoms. Keep in mind that interest/arousal disorder, orgasmic disorder, and pain/penetration disorders are all interconnected, so a lot of women have a combination of these issues. Therefore, I recommend that you take all the quizzes.

I created these abbreviated quizzes using information from the *Diagnostic and Statistical Manual of Mental Disorders*, 5th edition (DSM-5). These quizzes should not be used to self-diagnose. Instead, if you think you may have sexual dysfunction, please discuss your results with a qualified healthcare professional to determine if you meet the criteria for a formal diagnosis.

Female Sexual Interest/Arousal Disorder Quiz

If your answer to these four questions is yes, you might have a form of sexual dysfunction called *female sexual interest/arousal disorder*:

	Yes	No

1. Are you experiencing an absence of, or significant decrease in, at least three of the following?

   - Interest in having sex ❏ ❏
   - Sexual fantasies or erotic thoughts ❏ ❏
   - Initiation of sexual activity and receptiveness to a partner's initiation ❏ ❏
   - Excitement or pleasure during approximately 75 percent or more of your sexual activity ❏ ❏
   - Interest or arousal in response to sexual or erotic cues (whether internal, external, verbal, written, or visual) ❏ ❏
   - Sensations (in genitals or other bodily areas) during sexual activity in at least 75 percent of sexual encounters ❏ ❏

2. Have those symptoms persisted for a minimum of six months? ❏ ❏

3. Are your symptoms so bothersome that they cause you distress? ❏ ❏

4. Is your healthcare practitioner certain that the sexual dysfunction *is not* attributable to a nonsexual mental disorder (such as depression); severe relationship distress (like domestic violence) or other significant stressors; the effects of starting, stopping, or changing the dosage of a substance or medication; or another medical reason? ❏ ❏

Note: In the past, a lack of desire was called *female hypoactive sexual desire disorder*, and a lack of arousal was called *female sexual arousal disorder*. However, since there's a lot of overlap between sexual interest and sexual arousal, they are now considered one disorder.

Female Orgasmic Disorder Quiz

If your answer to these four questions is yes, you might have a form of sexual dysfunction called *female orgasmic disorder*.

	Yes	No
1. Have you noticed a significant delay in, infrequency of, or absence of orgasm *or* markedly reduced intensity of orgasmic sensations?	❑	❑
2. Have those symptoms occurred in approximately 75 percent or more of your sexual encounters during the past six months or more?	❑	❑
3. Are your symptoms so bothersome that they cause you distress?	❑	❑
4. Is your healthcare practitioner certain that the sexual dysfunction *is not* attributable to a nonsexual mental disorder (such as depression); severe relationship distress (like domestic violence) or other significant stressors; the effects of starting, stopping, or changing the dosage of a substance or medication; or another medical reason?	❑	❑

Genito-Pelvic Pain/Penetration Disorder Quiz

If your answer to these four questions is yes, you might have a form of sexual dysfunction called *genito-pelvic pain/penetration disorder*:

	Yes	No
1. Have you had persistent or recurrent difficulties with one or more of the following?		

- Vaginal penetration during intercourse ❏ ❏
- Vulvar, vaginal, or pelvic pain during attempts at intercourse or penetration ❏ ❏
- Fear or anxiety about vulvar, vaginal, or pelvic pain before, during, or after vaginal penetration ❏ ❏
- A lot of tensing or tightening of the pelvic-floor muscles during attempted vaginal penetration

2. Have these symptoms persisted for a minimum of six months? ❏ ❏

3. Are your symptoms so bothersome that they cause you distress? ❏ ❏

4. Is your healthcare practitioner certain that the sexual dysfunction *is not* attributable to a nonsexual mental disorder (such as depression); severe relationship distress (like domestic violence) or other significant stressors; the effects of starting, stopping, or changing the dosage of a substance or medication; or another medical reason? ❏ ❏

Other Specified Sexual Dysfunction and Other Unspecified Sexual Dysfunction Quiz

If you don't fit into one of the other sexual dysfunction categories and you answer yes to the following question, you might have *other specified sexual dysfunction* or *other unspecified sexual dysfunction*:

	Yes	No
1. Do you experience distressing symptoms typical of a sexual dysfunction that do not meet the criteria of one of the defined categories above?	❑	❑

Note: The major difference between other specified sexual dysfunction and other unspecified sexual dysfunction is whether your healthcare practitioner gives a specific reason that the symptoms described do not meet the criteria for one of the other classes.

Practical (Medicine-Free) Solutions That Actually Work

If your doctor confirms that you have sexual dysfunction, or if you don't technically have sexual dysfunction but you still want to know how to make your sex life even better, I'm a big believer in starting with low-risk, high-reward treatment options that don't involve unnecessary medication. With the exception of treatment for vaginal dryness or systemic hormones for menopause-related symptoms, I recommend considering these tips before starting a medication for sexual dysfunction.

Although transgender individuals and multiple-partner relationships are not specifically addressed, many of the following suggestions are likely to be applicable.

Address mismatched libidos (communication is crucial)

As Dr. Jess O'Reilly, host of the podcast *Sex with Dr. Jess*, pointed out during an interview she did, if you think about it, it's not surprising that a lot of couples have mismatched libidos. Just as people don't eat the same meals, in the same quantity, at the same time as another person, you can't expect to want exactly what your partner wants sexually. So if you and your partner are struggling to find a balance that doesn't leave one person feeling sexually exhausted and the other person feeling sexually deprived, know that you're not alone. This is one of the most common sexual issues that couples face. But if you try to ignore it, you'll probably end up with one or both partners having hurt feelings, frustration, and/or resentment.

Here are two of my favorite tips when it comes to dealing with mismatched libidos. The first tip comes from Dr. Jess.[2]

Tip 1: Come to a compromise.

To do this, first you need to know how far off your desired numbers are. (Hint: A lot of times, your numbers are closer than you think.) To figure this out, you and your partner should each take a sheet of paper and write down how often you want to have sex. Do you want it once a week, four times a week, or with every meal? Then, at the bottom of the paper, write down how often you perceive your partner to want sex. Do they want it once every other week or once per fiscal year?

Next, exchange papers and have a conversation to help you understand what the other person wants and find common ground. During your conversation, don't use shame, blame, or guilt to get your point across, and don't try to force them to make their sexual desire level match yours. Instead, both of you will need to be willing to make some relationship, behavior, and attitude changes to make the common ground work. And have realistic expectations — the probability of meeting exactly at the halfway point is low. Also, remember that neither person is right or wrong. Wanting more sex doesn't make a person a pervert, and wanting less sex doesn't make a person a prude.

Once you agree on a desired number, implementing the next suggestion will maximize the odds that you'll reach your goal.

Tip 2: Understand each other's sexual initiation style.

Simply stated, your sexual initiation style is what ignites your spontaneous or responsive desire. Do you want your partner to kiss you passionately or tease you? Romance you or talk dirty to you? Gently hug you or push you against the wall? Lots of people assume they know their partner's style, but research shows that many people have only some idea about what works for their partner. So I recommend that you google "sexual initiation style quiz" and each of you independently take a free online quiz. Then, share your results with each other.

In many cases a higher-desire partner will initiate sex in a way that is not at all appealing to the lower-desire partner. For instance, if someone wants to be romanced, but their partner is always talking dirty, that isn't gonna work. Their sexual requests will be DOA (dead on arrival). Not necessarily because their partner doesn't want sex, but because they don't want sex the way the higher-desire partner initiated it. So understanding your partner's initiation preferences can make or break your chances for sex.

If you try to have a conversation but it doesn't go very well, or if the thought of having this (or any other sexually related) conversation with your partner makes you want to crawl out of your skin, consider my next suggestion.

Talk it out (in therapy)

When I tell patients with a hormonal imbalance that they need to see a doctor with special training in managing hormones, they say, "No problem." When I tell patients who are snoring that they need to see a sleep specialist, they say, "No problem." But when I tell patients that they should consider therapy, a lot of them give me the "I'll think about it, doc" look. And if I specifically mention the potential benefits of seeing a sex therapist or a sex educator, I mostly get "I'm gonna pass; what else ya got?" looks. But whether you are dealing with sexual issues like mismatched libidos or other factors that are known to have a negative impact on people's sex lives, like stress, body-image issues, depression, anxiety, past sexual trauma, or current relationship issues, therapy can be incredibly beneficial.

Your doctor can help you figure out which type of therapy would be most appropriate for you. For instance, if you and your partner keep having the same fight, or if you're having a hard time communicating for any reason, couples therapy can be extremely helpful.

If dysfunctional beliefs are standing between you and the sex life you deserve, group-based or couples-based cognitive-behavioral therapy can help you dig into your subconscious to identify those issues. And if you were physically, emotionally, or sexually abused, you are likely to benefit from a trauma-informed psychotherapeutic approach.

If your doctor thinks a sex therapist or a sex educator would be helpful for you, please don't knock this idea until you really understand it. These individuals are not creepy people who want to meet you in a dark basement to talk about sex. They are trained professionals who can really help you get your sex life on track. For instance, in one study, 65 percent of 365 couples undergoing sex therapy for a range of sexual dysfunctions described their treatment as successful. That means

6.5 study participants out of 10 walked away with a better sex life! If you do an internet search for "American Association of Sexuality Educators, Counselors, and Therapists," or "Society for Sex Therapy and Research," you'll get a list of certified individuals. Their services are frequently covered by insurance.

Don't yuck your yum (have yourself some fun, sis)

One day I heard Shan Boodram, sexologist and host of a popular (and very relatable) podcast called *Lovers and Friends*, talking about how she never wants to "yuck someone else's yum." Sexually speaking, that means her goal is to be supportive of different sexual limits or boundaries. Whether someone is down for just about anything, they fall in the middle by drawing a line somewhere around armpit sex (which is surprisingly popular), or they say no to anything that doesn't happen in the missionary position with the lights off, Shan wants to make them feel comfortable as she educates them and they explore their sexuality.

That conversation made me think about patients who actually yuck *their own* yum.

To be clear, I'm not telling you what to like or what not to like, but I am suggesting that you have an honest conversation with yourself (and your partner, if you have one) about how far you'd like to go sexually. For some couples, an ideal sex life involves showing up in matching red flannel PJs every Thursday night for seven minutes of fun...missionary style. That's their yum. And there is absolutely, positively nothing wrong with that. But there are a lot of women who know what they want and how they want it (or they at least know what they want to try), but usually due to sociocultural beliefs or a fear of being judged or rejected by their partner, they don't voice their desires. They have been pleasure-shamed into yucking their own yum, even though the thought of their sex life makes them yawn.

Also, don't feel bad about fantasizing. Some women are reluctant to let their imaginations run wild because they start to feel a sense of guilt or shame, but they shouldn't. Some things that arouse you psychologically wouldn't arouse you in real life. In other words, just because you fantasize about something doesn't mean you want to actually carry out the fantasy. In fact, in most cases our fantasies wouldn't actually give us pleasure if we were to act on them. For instance, you might love to fantasize about bondage, but you might not actually enjoy being strapped to a table with a ball gag in your mouth in real life. Even if you fantasize about something like having sex with Dracula while the alien from the *E.T.* movie tells you what to do and how to do it, don't assume you have a deep, underlying character flaw. Fantasies don't have to mesh with real-life ethics or beliefs.

Just in case you're curious about what other people fantasize about, as reported in the *Journal of Sexual Medicine*, in a study called "What Exactly Is an Unusual Sexual Fantasy?" researchers looked at 1,516 people. Here is an excerpt from their findings:[3]

Female fantasies	Presence of fantasy (%)
Atmosphere and location are important in my sexual fantasies.	86.4
I have fantasized about having sex in a romantic location (e.g., on a deserted beach).	84.9
I have fantasized about having sex in an unusual place (e.g., in the office; public toilets).	81.7
I have fantasized about taking part in fellatio/cunnilingus. (Fellatio is oral stimulation of the penis. Cunnilingus is oral stimulation of female genitalia.)	78.5
I have fantasized about giving fellatio.	72.1

I have fantasized about being masturbated by my partner.	71.4
I have fantasized about having sex with someone I know who is not my spouse.	66.3
I have fantasized about masturbating my partner.	68.1
I have fantasized about being dominated sexually.	64.6
I have fantasized about making love openly in a public place.	57.3
I have fantasized about having sex with two men.	56.5
I have fantasized about being tied up by someone in order to obtain sexual pleasure.	52.1
I have fantasized about watching two women make love.	42.4
I have fantasized about my partner ejaculating on me.	41.3
I have fantasized about being masturbated by an unknown person.	33.4
I have fantasized about having sex with more than three people, both men and women.	30.9
I have fantasized about indulging in sexual swinging with a couple I do not know.	26.9

If you're looking for ideas to spice things up, Google "yes, no, maybe sex list." Then, after filling your lists out independently, you and your partner can compare answers (without coercion or judgment). If you are having a hard time discussing sexual desires or fantasies with your partner, a therapist can help you with effective communication. Even couples who are great at communicating about other issues can have a difficult time talking about sex.

Schedule maintenance sex
(because "tomorrow sex" rarely comes)

Some people think that scheduling sex isn't sexy. But nothing is sexier or says "I value this relationship" more than a woman choosing to show up and be ready and willing to have her responsive desire ignited instead of going to sleep or bingeing a show on Netflix after she's been working, taking care of kids, or just being an adult in general. But here's the catch: Ladies, when you show up, don't bring just your body. You also have to bring your mind and practice "mindful sex."

During mindful sex, your brain is focused on appreciating the wonderful experience taking place. Nothing else matters. It's not time to think about how your thighs look, how much you hate your boss, or random stuff like how much you love tacos. All your brainpower is going toward enjoying what is happening in the moment. You feel each touch and kiss. You appreciate every loving, passionate, or kinky glance. Your number one concern is sexual pleasure.

Focusing on the moment during intercourse sounds like pretty simple advice, but it's actually hard for a lot of people to stop their mind from wandering during sex. Making that change can take some practice. But that's OK! The good news is that if you practice mindfulness while you are doing everyday activities, you'll be better at it when you're having sex! For example, when you are brushing your teeth, focus on the taste of the toothpaste, the feeling of the bristles on your teeth, and the feeling of the water in your mouth. Or when you are eating, focus on the taste and feel of your food as you chew. If you immerse yourself in various moments during your daily routine and let your senses take over as you focus only on what is happening in each moment, it will be easier for you to immerse yourself during sex.

If you notice your mind drifting off to a nonsexual place during sex, just take a deep breath and consciously bring it back to the moment. But if your mind keeps wandering because the sex is boring or because your relationship is not in a good place, circle back to the tips from earlier in this chapter.

And if your mind is never available for sex because you are too stressed about life, work, and/or kids, talk to your partner. They should support you in ways that will alleviate your stress, but if they're not doing that, put it on your "We need to talk to the therapist about this" list.

Do a health and meds check-in (make sure you're in tip-top shape for the festivities)

Ask your healthcare practitioner to review your medications and your medical history. Below is a list of some common culprits that disrupt people's sex lives. In some cases, sexual problems will be improved by diagnosing and treating an underlying medical problem or by adjusting your treatment regimen to minimize sexual side effects.

Common medical issues/reasons for problems with sexual interest, arousal, and/or orgasms

- Anxiety disorder*
- Diabetes
- Depression*
- Endometriosis
- Fatigue
- Female genital mutilation
- Fibroids
- Hypertension (high blood pressure)
- Hyper- or hypothyroidism
- Hysterectomy

- Vaginal dryness due to menopause or perimenopause
- Medications like certain antidepressants, antianxiety meds, antihypertensives, histamine blockers, and hormonal medication
- Negative attitude toward sex or negative cultural conditioning (for example, believing that "respectable women" don't enjoy sex)
- Negative body image / being self-critical
- Neurologic conditions
- Pelvic organ prolapse (when one or more pelvic organs slip down from their normal position and bulge in the vagina)
- Pregnancy-related factors (pregnancy, trauma caused during delivery, adjustment to motherhood, vaginal dryness from breastfeeding)
- Relationship drama (like hostility toward your spouse)
- Stress*
- Substance abuse
- Traumatic sexual experiences (such as sexual abuse)
- Urinary incontinence (accidental bladder leakage)

   * Stress, depression, and anxiety cause some people to desire sex more, but those people tend to have lower levels of arousal/orgasm.

Embrace the dual-control model (sometimes, new lingerie isn't the answer)

In the introduction to this chapter, I told you about Katrina and all the things she tried in order to improve her sex life. But nothing she tried worked because she was focused on the wrong question. She thought the key to sexual ecstasy was figuring out what turned her on. But like many women, she forgot to ask a question that's often even more important: "What is turning me *off*, and what can I do about it?"

The sexy lingerie and all that other stuff was helpful, but it was never going to give Katrina the sex life she was looking for. If Katrina wanted to jump-start her libido, boost her sexual arousal, and maximize her sexual pleasure, she needed to understand a simple but powerful concept called the dual-control model.

The dual-control model, which is based on research by Erick Janssen and John Bancroft at the Kinsey Institute, is all about maximizing the number of things that excite you sexually and minimizing the number of things standing in the way of that goal.[4] The rules are pretty simple: The more things that turn you on, the more you want/enjoy sex. The more things that turn you off, the less you want/enjoy sex. If you have too many turnoffs (because you're stressed, you're worrying that sex might be painful, you feel that your partner can't be trusted, or you are dealing with unresolved trauma from sexual abuse), no amount of lingerie, candles, or sex toys that "guarantee a good time" will make you desire sex, get you aroused, or allow you to experience the level of sexual pleasure you're capable of having. It's a simple but powerful concept.

Medical Options

The main predictors of sexual satisfaction are physical health, psychological health, and the quality of the relationship. So the lifestyle suggestions listed earlier in this chapter work really well for a lot of people. But if the suggestions listed above (including therapy) don't resolve your issue(s) and your practitioner doesn't have any additional medicine-free tips that might work for you, medication is another option. However, be aware that aside from medications used to treat symptoms due to low estrogen (for example, menopausal hormone therapy or vaginal estrogen), the meds currently available for female sexual dysfunction have limited effectiveness. And, of course, all medications are associated with side effects and potential risks.

Female sexual interest/arousal disorder treatment options

*   **Testosterone.** No form of androgens (including testosterone) is Food and Drug Administration (FDA) approved to treat sexual interest and arousal disorders. However, some postmenopausal women find it helpful. For premenopausal women, we don't have enough scientific evidence to recommend for or against this treatment option for interest/arousal disorder. Due to the risks associated with fetal exposure, a woman shouldn't get pregnant while using testosterone.

    Short-term use of *transdermal testosterone* can be considered in postmenopausal women who understand the potential risks, which may be irreversible. These risks include hirsutism (abnormal growth of hair on a person's face and body), acne, and virilization (including clitoral enlargement and voice deepening). Female testosterone users should also be aware that most studies have not evaluated use past six months. Therefore, the long-term effects are unknown. For example, we don't know how testosterone use impacts breast cancer risk or other cancer risk.

    If you decide to try transdermal testosterone, have blood drawn to check a baseline testosterone level, then repeat the lab work after 3 to 6 weeks of initial use to ensure levels remain within the normal range for reproductive-aged women. If your desire level doesn't go up after you've been using it for six months, you should stop the medication. If you decide to proceed with ongoing therapy, get your testosterone levels checked every three to six months to make sure your levels aren't too high. You should also have blood drawn to monitor your lipids and liver function, and you should have annual mammograms.

Testosterone is available in other forms besides transdermal, but data are limited, and the Endocrine Society and the North American Menopause Society do not currently support their use.

- **Bupropion.** This medication is FDA approved to treat depression and assist with smoking cessation. For women who have female sexual dysfunction that is caused by their selective serotonin reuptake inhibitor (SSRI) antidepressant, adding bupropion to their medication regimen may improve desire, arousal, and orgasmic dysfunction, but this is an off-label use. Potential side effects include insomnia, anxiety, and high blood pressure.

- **Bremelanotide.** This medication was approved by the FDA in 2019 for low desire in premenopausal women. But in a study of 1,247 women, it was found that there was no significant difference in the number of satisfying sexual events, although some women did report increased sexual desire. This medication is administered as a subcutaneous injection at least forty-five minutes before anticipated sexual activity. Common side effects include nausea (mostly with the first injection), vomiting, flushing, and headaches. And 1 percent of women experienced possibly permanent hyperpigmentation of the face, breasts, and gums. Women with high blood pressure or heart problems should not take bremelanotide.

- **Flibanserin.** The FDA rejected this medicine twice because of concerns regarding effectiveness and safety. In

2015 the FDA approved it for premenopausal women with low sexual desire. However, the overall quality of evidence for effectiveness was very low. The average improvement is less than one additional satisfying sexual event a month. This medication is taken by mouth daily. Side effects include dizziness, sleepiness, nausea, and fatigue. Alcohol must be avoided.

- **Estrogen.** Vaginal estrogen can be used to treat vaginal dryness. Or if a woman with a previously satisfying sex life presents with sexual problems that started with the onset of hot flashes, night sweats, sleep disruption, and resulting fatigue, treatment of menopausal symptoms with oral postmenopausal hormone therapy may lead to improvement in the sexual problem. However, in the absence of menopausal symptoms, oral estrogen with or without progestin has not been shown to specifically improve sexual satisfaction. So oral estrogen (or estrogen plus progestin) should not be used for the sole purpose of improving sexual satisfaction.

- **Over-the-counter herbal supplements.** Many women are interested in trying supplements to increase sexual desire and pleasure, but they haven't been proven to improve sexual function more than a placebo ("sugar pill") does. Furthermore, due to the limited number of well-designed studies and the lack of oversight when it comes to the production of herbal supplements, some available options may be unsafe. If you choose to use an herbal supplement, please proceed with caution.

Female orgasmic disorder treatment options

Orgasmic disorders can be lifelong or they can start later in life, and they can be situational (meaning they occur only in some situations) or generalized (they occur all the time). An example of situational orgasmic dysfunction is being able to have an orgasm during masturbation but not with a partner.

In an effort to treat orgasmic dysfunction (or add more oomph to their existing orgasms), some people get G-spot injections, clitoral-hood reduction, and other vaginal rejuvenation procedures. However, the American College of Obstetricians and Gynecologists (a reputable organization that supports evidence-based medicine) states that these procedures "are not medically indicated, pose substantial risk, and their safety and effectiveness have not been established."[5] Additionally, although your doctor may recommend a medication for an off-label use, no meds have shown convincing evidence of effectiveness when it comes to treating orgasmic dysfunction. No supplements have been proven to work either. So treatment mostly consists of education, counseling/therapy, and the use of devices like vibrators.

We need more large clinical trials to determine the best treatment recommendations for female orgasmic disorder. Therefore, suggestions may vary greatly from practitioner to practitioner. Here's a brief overview of some options that may be considered after ensuring that a medical issue, social issue, or medication isn't the culprit:

Treatment for people who have never had an orgasm

Treatment usually starts with a clinician educating a woman about her anatomy and having a frank discussion with her about the adequacy of stimulation that she receives. Also, individual or couples talk therapy is frequently an important part of the process. For example, a therapist can help a couple work through relationship problems or dispel negative beliefs about sex. Additionally, "directed masturbation" (sometimes known as masturbation training) is a first-line therapy for women who have never experienced an orgasm. During these training sessions, women are taught how to reach orgasm through self-stimulation. Once the person becomes orgasmic regularly, if they have a partner, the partner is brought into the session so that they can learn to bring their previously nonorgasmic partner to orgasm. Some patients need more or less assistance, but having weekly or twice weekly sessions for six to eight weeks has a great success rate.

As an alternative to directed masturbation, you can use a self-help guide, but directed masturbation has much better results. If you proceed with self-help, clitoral vacuum suction devices or vibrators work well because they increase clitoral blood flow. If you don't feel comfortable going to an adult toy store, you can buy a vibrator at many chain pharmacies — they are usually in the section with moisturizers and lubricants. You can also order one online. (In 2000, the FDA approved a battery-powered clitoral suction device intended to improve arousal and orgasm by increasing blood flow and engorgement. However, at this time, its advantages over other over-the-counter vibrators are not clear.) *Becoming Orgasmic: A Sexual and Personal Growth Program for Women*, revised and expanded edition, by Joseph LoPiccolo and Julia Heiman, is an excellent self-help manual.

If a patient avoids sex because of anxiety, exposure therapy may be incorporated. With exposure therapy, the patient is slowly exposed to whatever causes their anxiety. For example, if someone becomes very anxious when they are nude in front of their partner, they slowly learn to overcome that feared experience. Clinicians may also recommend that couples proceed with sensate focus exercises, which are all about learning to touch and be touched. Sensate focus exercises usually begin by having partners exchange pleasurable touch of areas of the body other than the genitals and breasts, and the couple gradually progresses to "sensual" intercourse.

Treatment for people who have had an orgasm

For women who have had orgasms before, the treatment strategy is not as straightforward. Treatments focus on the cause of the dysfunction by looking for physical, psychological, and interpersonal causes. That process may involve a number of people, including a cognitive-behavioral therapist and/or a sex therapist. Even if you've had orgasms before, *Becoming Orgasmic* is an excellent book to consider.

For people who have never had an orgasm as well as people who have stopped having orgasms, the president of the American Association of Sexuality Educators, Counselors, and Therapists (AASECT), Dr. Rosalyn Dischiavo, recommends *The Body Keeps the Score* by Bessel van der Kolk and *Pleasure Activism: The Politics of Feeling Good* by adrienne maree brown.

Genito-pelvic pain/penetration disorder (aka pain with sex) treatment options

Nearly 3 out of 4 women have pain during intercourse at some time during their lives. For some women, the pain is only a temporary problem, but for others, it's a long-term problem. There are lots of causes for pain with sex. Although discussing each one of them goes beyond the scope of this book, table 1 lists some of the common culprits. After the table, I'll go into detail about two important causes that are frequently overlooked. Some of the other issues are discussed in part 2 of the book.

Note that telling your practitioner when you experience the pain will help them determine the exact cause.

Table 1. Some Causes of Sexual Pain

Type/location of pain	Possible causes

Pain at the entrance of the vagina during initial penetration	• Decreased lubrication
	  ○ Hormonal contraception
	  ○ Decreased vaginal arousal
	• Low estrogen
	  ○ Breastfeeding
	  ○ Medications (such as certain birth control)
	  ○ Menopause/perimenopause (see chapter 14)
	  ○ Postpartum
	• Constriction or obstruction of the vaginal opening
	  ○ Chemotherapy or radiation
	  ○ Childbirth
	  ○ Congenital anomaly
	  ○ Inflammation, infection, or a skin disorder
	  ○ Pelvic organ prolapse (when one or more pelvic organs slip down from their normal position and bulge into the vagina; see spotlight on p. 287)
	  ○ Scarring from pelvic surgery
	  ○ Tight pelvic-floor muscles
	  ○ Vaginismus (see p. 69)
	  ○ Female genital cutting

Table 1. Some Causes of Sexual Pain (continued)

Type/location of pain	Possible causes
Pain with deep thrusting	• Endometriosis (when tissue that is similar to the inside lining of the uterus, or endometrium, is found outside the uterus; see spotlight on p. 163) • Uterine fibroids (noncancerous growths in the wall of the uterus; see spotlight on p. 196) • Ovarian cysts (see p. 175) • Pelvic inflammatory disease (see p. 302) • Tight pelvic-floor muscles • Retroverted uterus (uterus is tilted backward)
Nonspecific/ general	• History of abuse • Relationship problems • Mental-health issues (such as depression or anxiety) • Chronic pelvic pain (pain in the area below your belly button and between your hips that lasts six months or longer) • Pelvic congestion syndrome (pain due to dilated veins in the pelvic area) • Bladder or gastrointestinal problems • Vulvodynia (see p. 70)

It is not normal to have pain during sex, so make sure you tell your practitioner about your discomfort. The best treatment will depend on the cause of your pain. You may need to involve an ob-gyn, sex counselor, physical therapist, pain specialist, psychologist, or another type of clinician.

Vaginismus

Vaginismus is the involuntary contracting or tensing of muscles around the vagina. This involuntary spasm happens when something is about to be put in the vagina, such as a tampon or a penis. For some women, the condition is mildly uncomfortable, but for others the pain is so severe that nothing can be put in the vagina.

We aren't sure why some people experience vaginismus, but it may be due to:

- anxiety
- childbirth injuries
- a medical procedure/surgery (such as a hysterectomy)
- fear of sex or negative feelings about sex (due to past sexual abuse)

It is possible to get vaginismus even if you've been able to enjoy penetration in the past.

To diagnose this condition, your practitioner will perform a pelvic exam to confirm the presence of muscle spasms. You can ask them to apply a topical numbing cream to the outside of your vagina before the exam to make the process more comfortable for you, and your practitioner should stop the exam if you ask them to.

If you are diagnosed with vaginismus, treatments will focus on reducing the involuntary muscle spasms. These may include the following:

- Pelvic-floor physical therapy is extremely helpful for a lot of patients. During sessions, a specially trained physical therapist will use a variety of methods to teach you how to relax your pelvic-floor muscles. (I recommend seeing a physical therapist who is certified by the American Physical Therapy Association.)
- Vaginal Botox injections (which are administered under local anesthesia or sedation) can also help.
- Your practitioner may also recommend that you use tube-shaped devices called vaginal dilators at home. Their primary purpose is to stretch the vagina. There isn't a lot of research on exactly how the dilators should be used in terms of timing, duration, or technique. I recommend that patients start with the smallest dilator and slowly work their way up. For example, you can start with five minutes, but after a while, you'll be able to insert the dilator into your vagina for ten or fifteen minutes. You can use numbing medicine when using the dilators so that they cause less discomfort.
- If there is a history of trauma, relationship issues, or anxiety, therapy may also be very beneficial to address factors that may be contributing to vaginismus.

Vulvodynia

Vulvodynia is diagnosed if someone has vulvar pain for at least three months and all other possible causes of pain are ruled out. This pain is most commonly described as burning, stinging, stabbing, irritation, or rawness. Some people also report aching, soreness, throbbing, or swelling. They may also notice pain during sex or when they attempt to insert a tampon. If the pain involves only the vestibule (which is the shallow depression between the labia minora that begins below the clitoris and contains the opening to the urethra and the vaginal opening), it's called *vestibulodynia*. When it's confined to the glans clitoris and clitoral hood, it's called *clitorodynia*. If the pain is widespread on the vulva, it's called *vulvodynia*. *Provoked vulvodynia* happens when the area is touched (for some people, even the touch of underwear or clothing can lead to pain). *Spontaneous vulvodynia* pain is constant, or it comes and goes without a known trigger.

Vulvodynia is likely caused by different factors working together. Some of these may include:

- damage or irritation of the nerves of the vulva
- inflammation of the vulva
- long-term reactions to certain infections (such as recurrent yeast infections)
- dysfunction of the muscles of the pelvic floor
- conditions that affect nearby muscles or bones

Before diagnosing you with vulvodynia, your practitioner will try to rule out other causes of vulvar pain, such as a yeast infection, vaginal dryness due to menopause, a skin condition, or vaginismus. Once other causes are excluded, the cotton swab test is frequently used to make the diagnosis. For this test, a cotton swab is used to touch different areas of the vulva. If you experience pain with no known underlying issues to explain the pain, a diagnosis of vulvodynia is considered.

If you are diagnosed with vulvodynia, you may have to try several different treatments before you find one that works. Options include:

- **Local anesthetics.** These can be used for extended periods, but a lot of patients also find it helpful to use local anesthetics for temporary symptom relief (e.g., applying lidocaine thirty minutes before sex). If you choose this option, your partner may also have temporary numbness after sexual contact.

- **Antidepressants and antiseizure drugs.** It can take a few weeks for these medications to work, but they sometimes help with the pain. Some antidepressants can be provided in the form of a cream that is applied to the skin.
- **Hormone creams.** In some cases, estrogen cream that's applied to the vulva may help relieve vulvodynia.
- **Physical therapy.** Physical therapy exercises can help relax the pelvic muscles.
- **Trigger point therapy.** A trigger point is a small area of tightly contracted muscle. Pain from a trigger point travels to nearby areas. During trigger point therapy, the tight area of muscle is massaged to relax it. Sometimes a combination of an anesthetic drug and a steroid are also injected into the trigger point to provide relief.
- **Nerve blocks.** A nerve block is a type of anesthesia in which an anesthetic drug is injected into the nerves that carry pain signals from the vulva to the spinal cord. Sometimes, Botox is used to relax muscles of the pelvic floor.
- **Surgery.** For some women with persistent localized pain that is confined to the vestibule, surgery to remove the affected skin and tissue (vestibulectomy) can relieve pain — of course, you'd need to understand the risks and benefits before the procedure.
- **Vulvar care.** The following vulvar care tips may help:
  - Clean the vulva with water only.
  - Wear 100 percent cotton underwear.
  - Use 100 percent cotton menstrual pads.
  - Use lubricants during sex, but don't select flavored lube or lubes with cooling/warming sensation.

- ○   Use cool gel packs on the vulva.
- ○   After you bathe, apply a thin layer of preservative-free oil or petroleum jelly to hold in moisture and protect the skin.
- **Talk therapy.** Talk therapy is recommended to help you deal with chronic pain. It is not being recommended because your pain is not real.

DR. NITA'S NOTE
Domestic Violence Spotlight

Maya Angelou once said, "When people show you who they are, believe them."[6] Truer words were never spoken. So if you're in a relationship, let's determine what your partner's actions are showing you about them. Be honest with yourself. Does your partner...[7]

- embarrass or mock you in front of friends or family?
- downplay your accomplishments?
- make you feel like you're unable to make decisions?
- use intimidation or threats to gain compliance?
- tell you you're nothing without them?
- treat you roughly — grab, push, pinch, or hit you?
- call you several times a night or show up to make sure you're where you said you would be?
- say hurtful things or abuse you and then blame it on drugs or alcohol?
- blame you for how they feel or act?
- pressure you sexually for things you aren't ready for?
- make you feel like there's no way out of the relationship?
- prevent you from doing things you want — like spending time with friends or family?

- try to keep you from leaving after a fight, or leave you somewhere after a fight, to "teach you a lesson"?

Do you...

- sometimes feel scared of how your partner may behave?
- frequently make excuses for your partner's behavior?
- believe that you could help your partner change if only you changed something about yourself?
- try not to do anything that would cause conflict or make your partner angry?
- always do what your partner wants you to do instead of what you want?
- stay with your partner because you're afraid of what they would do if you broke up?

If you answered yes to some of these questions, which are all signs of domestic abuse (sometimes called *intimate partner violence* or *domestic violence*), it's important for you to acknowledge the fact that you're being abused. Domestic abuse, which impacts 1 in 3 women worldwide,[8] can be emotional, physical, sexual, or economic in nature.

Emotional abuse, which frequently masquerades as healthy behaviors, can be particularly hard to recognize. In fact, in many emotionally abusive relationships, the person fails to realize the harm their partner is causing and may even love them more for it. For example, you may interpret your partner's demanding actions as caring. But there's a difference between being cared for and being controlled. Emotional abuse leaves scars you can't see, and it's often a precursor to physical abuse.

Physical abuse is when a person hurts or tries to hurt a partner by using some type of force, such as shoving, slapping, pinching, or using physical restraint. Even if the encounter ends without any physical proof such as cuts or bruises, these scenarios still constitute abuse.

Sexual abuse is nonconsensual sexual contact. Examples include coerced nudity or unwanted touching or sexual intercourse. And, to be clear, no matter how many times you've said yes in the past, any nonconsensual sexual contact is considered a violation. This even pertains to spouses. If a married person forces their spouse to have sex with them, that's marital rape. If you tell someone you don't want to be touched, they should take their hands off you as quickly as they would drop a ball of hot lava, no questions asked. And being unable to give consent — because you're drunk or high, for example — is the same as saying no.

Economic abuse involves controlling someone financially. The abuser restricts access to money or attempts to keep the abused from working or going to school. The choice between staying in the abusive relationship and poverty or even homelessness often leaves the abused person feeling trapped.

If you're not sure if you're being abused, or if you know you're experiencing abuse but you're unsure of how to safely leave the relationship, domestic abuse advocates can help you determine your best next steps. Leaving an abusive relationship, and just before leaving, can be a dangerous time. It's important that you devise a safe exit plan.

To reach an advocate at the National Domestic Violence Hotline, call 1-800-799-SAFE (7233), go to thehotline.org, or text "START" to 88788. You can also research local resources. No matter what option you choose, be mindful of the ways that your abuser may track your actions — for instance, they may monitor your phone bills or internet history.

In preparing to leave an abusive relationship, remember:

- Abuse isn't your fault.
- No one deserves to be abused.

- You're fabulous, and you deserve to be loved accordingly.

  Don't ignore the truth when an abuser shows you who they truly are, no matter how much you love them. Trust patterns; don't trust apologies.

Reclaiming Sexual Pleasure

Many women who think they have sexual dysfunction actually don't. Instead, they have unresolved relationship issues or, like many women, they have trouble communicating their sexual desires. Another big culprit is monotony. For example, if their partner always inserts his penis at the same angle, and his thrusting is always on beat with the happy birthday song, it might not be that they don't want to have sex, but rather that they just don't want to have *that* kind of sex. That's not sexual dysfunction. That's boredom.

However, if you're concerned about sexual dysfunction, the only way you'll know for sure is if you discuss your symptoms with a healthcare practitioner who is qualified to properly diagnose you. If you do in fact have sexual dysfunction, your practitioner should be willing and able to help you determine your best next steps. And even if you don't technically have sexual dysfunction, they should be willing to address your sexual concerns.

Many healthcare practitioners lack adequate knowledge and training in the diagnosis and management of female sexual dysfunction. Therefore, if you don't feel as though you are getting the level of care you desire, get a second opinion.

Chapter 5

Grown Folks' Sex Ed

Sexually Transmitted Infections and Diseases

Once, a guy told his three girlfriends to meet him in the parking lot of my ob-gyn clinic. Then he proceeded to "politely" introduce them to each other and tell them they all needed to get tested for syphilis (which he suspected he got from a *fourth* lover). Just in case you're wondering, the meet and greet did not go well...

Then there was the time I spent my afternoon at an assisted-living facility, testing the residents for gonorrhea and chlamydia. To make a long story short, after a little detective work, we figured out that patient zero was a very busy eighty-year-old with a big bottle of little blue pills.

I could also talk about the hands I've held and tears I've wiped because of infertility struggles caused by a past sexually transmitted disease. Or I could tell you about the time I had to tell a newly divorced, middle-aged, single mom who had recently started having a little dating-app fun that she had contracted HIV. Then we could go on to discuss the disappointingly high number of times I've had to tell a married woman that she has a sexually transmitted infection and have her sincerely ask, "But I'm married. How did I get it?"

I could go on … and on, from the minivan-driving soccer mom to the Gucci-wearing woman with a ridiculous number of zeros in her bank account, the high school valedictorian, or the Amish woman who arrived for her appointment in a horse and carriage. In other words, it doesn't matter who you are or where you come from — sexually transmitted infections are willing and able to infect you. *No one* — and I truly mean *no one* — is immune to getting one. You may think you're the exception to that rule, but unless you've sworn off vaginal, anal, and oral sex as well as any genital skin-to-skin contact, I assure you that you are not. I wish this wasn't the case, but I'm sure at some point in my career, I've diagnosed a person leading a life similar to yours with an STD.

That said, this chapter is not about moralizing or judging. I'm only interested in empowering women to take control of their sexual health. And part of that job means letting women know that STDs are common and that there are lots of great treatment options. But prevention and protection should be every sexually active person's mantra.

Staying Safe While Having Fun: Practical Questions and Answers about STDs

Even if you're sure that your sexual well-being is safe and sound in your monogamous relationship, I guarantee you that somebody you know could benefit from the info in this chapter. Maybe sharing what you read will help your teenager who is going off to college, one of your single friends, your widowed mother, or your Uncle Joe, who spends a suspicious amount of time at his neighbor's house "unclogging pipes."

To keep it simple, I'll give you the answers to practical

questions that anyone who is sexually active should know about. After you've finished reading this chapter, you'll be in a good position to protect yourself, and if you *do* find yourself with an STD, you'll know what to do.

Question 1: I thought they were all sexually transmitted diseases (STDs). Why am I seeing the term *sexually transmitted infections* (STIs), and what's the difference?

Think of an infection as the first step on the road to a disease. When a sexually transmitted pathogen like bacteria (such as chlamydia or gonorrhea), virus (such as herpes), or parasite (such as trichomoniasis) enters your body, you have a sexually transmitted *infection*. Once the infection is in your body, two things can happen:

- If the pathogen is able to multiply enough to disrupt normal body functions or damage structures in the body (in other words, cause medical issues), your STI has officially become a sexually transmitted *disease*.
- If the infection goes away on its own or with treatment without causing any health problems, it remains a sexually transmitted *infection*.

For example, let's say you're infected with the human papillomavirus (HPV):

- If the HPV infection multiplies and gives you genital warts, the HPV is considered a sexually transmitted *disease*.
- If the HPV infection goes away without causing any health problems, the HPV is considered a sexually transmitted *infection*.

So while some health organizations use the terms interchangeably, technically STIs and STDs are different. All STDs start out as STIs, and the term *STD* suggests a more serious problem.

Question 2: You mentioned that sexually transmitted infections are common; exactly how common are we talking?

The short answer is *very*. But here is a more detailed answer: About one in five people in the United States have an STI on any given day. So at this very moment, over 60 million people in the US are walking around with an STI. To put that into perspective, the next time you're in a meeting or at the grocery store, look at five people around you. Statistically speaking, one of them has a sexually transmitted infection. That's a lot of people.

And please don't make the mistake of thinking you're too old to get an STI. Yes, it's true that people aged fifteen to twenty-four get almost half of the 26 million or so new STIs that are diagnosed each year, but when you run the numbers, you are still left with millions and millions of STIs to go around. This is why the AARP (formerly known as the American Association of Retired Persons) recently released articles to warn their members about the increase in STI rates for older adults.

Question 3: What sexually transmitted infections should I look out for if I have vaginal or anal sex?

Table 2 lists some common STIs that pop up over and over — *and over* — in clinics and hospitals around the world, though these are not all the STIs under the sun. You'll notice that in a lot of cases, people with STIs/STDs won't notice any symptoms. In one study it was found that only 10 percent of men and 5 to 30 percent of women with chlamydia developed symptoms.[1] So the only way you can know for sure if you have an STI or STD is to get tested. It's important to remember this because even if you don't notice a single symptom, some STDs can still cause long-term complications (such as infertility or pelvic pain). While the table below lists many possible signs and symptoms, please note that some less-common ones may not be included. Also, having an STI changes the cells lining the vagina, penis, rectum, and mouth. So if you have an infection like chlamydia or gonorrhea, that makes it easier to contract another, like HIV.[2]

Table 2. Common STDs and Their Symptoms

Sexually transmitted disease (STD)	Possible signs, symptoms, and complications of vaginal, urinary tract, anal, or rectal infections in females
Bacterial	
Chlamydia (aka "the clam")	• Often no symptoms • Yellow or clear discharge from the vagina or urethra • Painful or frequent urination • Vaginal bleeding between periods • Long-term abdominal or pelvic pain • Rectal bleeding, discharge, or pain • May cause a reaction throughout the body known as reactive arthritis. This can lead to joint pain, pink eye, and/or a rash • Infertility • Ectopic pregnancy (pregnancy outside the uterus)

Table 2. Common STDs and Their Symptoms (continued)

Sexually transmitted disease (STD)	Possible signs, symptoms, and complications of vaginal, urinary tract, anal, or rectal infections in females
Gonorrhea (aka "the clap" or "the drip")	• Often no symptoms or very mild ones • Yellow or greenish discharge from the vagina or urethra • Painful or frequent urination • Vaginal bleeding between periods • Long-term abdominal or pelvic pain • Rectal bleeding, discharge, or pain • Can spread through the body, causing problems such as joint pain, a rash, or heart problems • Infertility • Ectopic pregnancy (pregnancy outside the uterus)
Syphilis (aka "the great imitator" or "the great pretender")	• Often symptoms that are too mild to notice • There are four stages of syphilis. During the primary stage, you might notice one or more painless genital ulcers. The sores typically last three to six weeks and go away even if you don't get treated. But even after the sores heal, treatment is needed to prevent progression to the other stages. (Later stages are discussed in question 16, p. 107).

Table 2. Common STDs and Their Symptoms (continued)

Sexually transmitted disease (STD)	Possible signs, symptoms, and complications of vaginal, urinary tract, anal, or rectal infections in females
Viral	
Genital herpes	• Sometimes symptoms that are too mild to notice • Burning, itching, or tingling where the virus first entered the body • Small red bumps or tiny white blisters or ulcers on the genitals, buttocks, thighs, or anus. Sores are typically painful and sometimes itchy, especially as they heal
Hepatitis B or **hepatitis C**	• Often no symptoms • Fever • Fatigue • Loss of appetite • Nausea/vomiting • Abdominal pain • Dark urine • Light-colored stool • Joint pain • Yellow skin or eyes (jaundice)
HIV	• Within 2 to 4 weeks after infection, most people have flulike symptoms (fever, chills, sore throat, muscle aches, fatigue). Since the symptoms are nonspecific, most people brush them off. After this, a decade or longer can pass with no symptoms.

Table 2. Common STDs and Their Symptoms (continued)

Sexually transmitted disease (STD)	Possible signs, symptoms, and complications of vaginal, urinary tract, anal, or rectal infections in females
High-risk human papillomavirus (HPV)	• Precancer or cancer in the anus/genital region • Usually resolves on its own without causing precancer or cancer
Low-risk human papillomavirus (HPV)	• Genital or anal warts that may be skin-colored or whitish • May resolve on its own without causing warts
Molluscum contagiosum	• Raised, round, skin-colored bumps, usually smaller than 6 millimeters wide, with a small dent at the top, near the center. In addition to being an STD, this can also be transmitted through sharing towels or skin-to-skin contact.
Parasitic	
Pubic lice (aka "crabs")	• Genital itching • Dark spots on the skin where pubic lice are living. These come from the crabs' bites. • Visible lice eggs (nits) or crawling lice
Trichomoniasis (aka "trich")	• Often no symptoms • Bad-smelling vaginal discharge that is white, gray, yellow, or green • Redness, burning, soreness, or itching of the genitals • Pain while peeing

Question 4: What are some of the STIs that can be transmitted if I receive or give oral sex?

See table 3 for a summary. We need more research to get a full understanding of how likely STI transmission is for some of these organisms during oral sex, but if a person with an infected throat, mouth, or lips performs oral sex on you, you may be at risk of getting chlamydia, gonorrhea, herpes, or HPV in your vagina, urinary tract, or anus/rectum. It is also possible to get syphilis when receiving oral sex from a partner with a syphilis sore or rash on the lips or mouth or in the throat. The risk of getting HIV while receiving oral sex on the vagina or anus from an infected partner is thought to be extremely low. If you get infected during oral sex, you will have the same signs and symptoms as the ones listed in table 2.

If you give oral sex, infections you can get include, but are not limited to, chlamydia, gonorrhea, herpes, and HPV in your mouth or throat. You can also get syphilis, hepatitis A, hepatitis B, or HIV, but the risk of getting HIV is low.

It is possible to have an STD in more than one area at the same time. For example, you can have an STD in the genitals and the throat. And you may not have symptoms at either location. That is why testing is so important.

Table 3. Oral Sex STDs and Their Symptoms

Sexually transmitted disease (STD)	Possible signs, symptoms, and complications of mouth/ throat infections
Bacterial	
Chlamydia	• Often no symptoms • Sore throat

Table 3. Oral Sex STDs and Their Symptoms (continued)

Sexually transmitted disease (STD)	Possible signs, symptoms, and complications of mouth/throat infections
Gonorrhea	• Often no symptoms • Sore throat • Might spread through the body causing joint pain, a rash, and/or heart problems
Syphilis	• Often no symptoms • Primary syphilis involves painless ulcers or sores on the lips, mouth, or throat. If not treated, the infection can progress to other stages of syphilis. See question 16 (p. 107) for details.
Viral	
Hepatitis A or **hepatitis B**	• Same as Hepatitis B or C symptoms listed in table 2
Oral herpes	• Often no symptoms • Cold sore(s)
HIV	• Same as symptoms listed in table 2
High-risk human papillomavirus (HPV)	• Precancer or cancer of the head and neck • May resolve on its own without causing precancer or cancer
Low-risk human papillomavirus (HPV)	• Warts in the throat that may cause changes in the voice, shortness of breath, or difficulty speaking • May resolve on its own without causing warts

Question 5: When it comes to HIV, which is riskiest: anal sex, vaginal sex, or oral sex?

Anal sex is the riskiest and oral sex is the least risky, with vaginal intercourse falling in the middle risk-wise.

The walls of the anus and rectum are thin, and they have a lot of blood vessels that can be injured during penetration. Also, the anus doesn't self-lubricate like the vagina does. Those factors make you more vulnerable to HIV and other STIs.[3] Using a male latex condom with lots and lots and lots of silicone- or water-based lubricant will keep the anal walls nice and slippery. Since that will reduce the chances of cuts and tears, you'll decrease your risk of getting or giving an STI during anal sex.[4] But even with plenty of lube, male condoms fail more often during anal sex than they do during vaginal or oral sex.

Tip: Unlike water-based lubes, silicone lubes don't evaporate quickly. Therefore, they are a great choice for anal sex.

Question 6: If I get an STI, when will I test positive, and when will symptoms show up?

The "window period" is the time between when a person gets a sexually transmitted infection and when a screening test can accurately detect the infection. (Screening tests are done to detect potential health problems or disease in people who do not have any symptoms of disease.) However, if a person knows they have been exposed to a sexually transmitted infection, they *should not* wait until the end of the window period to see a healthcare practitioner. Sometimes, the doctor will treat a patient based on their exposure, even though they don't have any symptoms or a positive test yet.

If you develop symptoms, the "incubation period" is the length of time between when you are infected and when your signs or symptoms appear. Table 4 lists average times, so you could see symptoms sooner or much later than these time frames. Additional information about HIV testing is included below the table.

One additional STI to be aware of: Mycoplasma genitalium is a type of bacteria that can cause symptoms such as vaginal discharge and irritation. Screening is not currently recommended in asymptomatic people, but in some cases (e.g., persistent symptoms), your practitioner may test you.

Table 4. STI Testing Guidelines

STI	Testing method/type	Window period	Incubation period
Chlamydia	Urine specimen or swab of vagina, rectum, or throat	1 week catches most; 2 weeks catches almost all	7–21 days
Gonorrhea	Urine specimen or swab of vagina, rectum, or throat	1 week catches most; 2 weeks catches almost all	1–14 days
Hepatitis B	Blood test, antibody testing method	3–6 weeks	60–180 days

Table 4. STI Testing Guidelines (continued)

STI	Testing method/type	Window period	Incubation period
Hepatitis C	Blood test, antibody testing method	2 months catches most; 6 months catches almost all	15–180 days
Herpes	Swab of lesion	Swab may be performed as soon as the first blister appears. Ideally, this test should be done within 48 hours of the appearance of the lesion (Accuracy of the test decreases as the lesion heals. If a scab is noted over the healing lesion, your clinician should attempt to remove the scab prior to swabbing it.)	2–12 days
	Blood test, antibody testing method	3–6 weeks catches most; 4 months catches almost all	2–12 days

Table 4. STI Testing Guidelines (continued)

STI	Testing method/ type	Window period	Incubation period
HIV	Nucleic acid test (blood drawn from a vein, not a finger prick)	10–33 days	14 days to years
	Antigen and antibody test performed in a lab on blood taken from a *vein*	18–45 days	
	Antigen and antibody test performed on blood taken from a *finger prick*	18–90 days	
	Antibody test (finger prick or oral fluid)	23–90 days	
High-risk HPV (cancer and precancer)	Pap test, HPV test, or both for women; screening not recommended for men	3 weeks to several years for women	Months to years
Low-risk HPV (genital/anal warts)	Screening not recommended for women or men		2 weeks to many months
Molluscum conta-giosum	No screening test		2 weeks to 6 months

Table 4. STI Testing Guidelines (continued)

STI	Testing method/ type	Window period	Incubation period
Pubic lice	No screening test		2–21 days
Syphilis	Blood test	1 month catches most; 3 months catches almost all	10–90 days
Trichomo- niasis	Swab of vagina	1 week catches most; 1 month catches almost all	5–28 days

HIV Testing

- If you think you've been exposed to HIV in the past seventy-two hours, your healthcare practitioner might recommend post-exposure prophylaxis (PEP) to help protect you from becoming HIV positive.
- HIV testing can be performed in different ways. A positive result must be confirmed with additional testing.
- **Standard tests.** Blood is taken from a vein and sent to the lab. Results are usually available in a few days. In general, tests that use blood from a vein can detect HIV sooner after infection than tests done with blood from a finger prick or with oral fluid.
- **Rapid tests.** This option uses blood from a finger prick or oral fluid. Test results only take five to forty minutes.
- **Home tests.** Home tests that require a finger prick are mailed to a lab, and the lab calls you with results. Another home test, OraQuick, uses oral fluids instead of blood. You get these results in twenty minutes.

Question 7: I'm trying to protect my body at all costs. If I'm willing to go full-court press with my STI questions, what should I ask someone before we have sex?

You should *always* ask the following seven questions — think of them as your "sex starter kit." But remember, they're just a starting point. If your intuition tells you to dig deeper and ask more questions … dig deeper. (And, of course, make sure you answer these same questions for your partner.)

a. When was the last time you had vaginal or anal sex with someone, or when was the last time you gave or received oral sex?

Yes, this is a personal question. But you are about to exchange bodily fluids with this person. From a medical standpoint, there is nothing more personal than that. Without the answer to this question, you can't assess your risk level.

b. When was the last time you got tested for STIs?

Now that you know all about window periods, you can determine if you feel comfortable with the timing. For example, if John gets chlamydia while having unprotected sex with Brenda on January 1st and he has an STI screening on January 3rd, his chlamydia test probably won't be positive yet.

Note: Currently, oral and anal/rectal STI screening is only routinely performed for men who have sex with men, but the CDC has recently expanded guidance to consider screening these sites for other people as well. If you or your partner is worried about an infection in the throat or anus/rectum, you should ask to be screened.

c. Which STIs were you tested for?

In appendix A, I've included a chart with official STI screening recommendations from the Centers for Disease Control (CDC). I recommend that you ask if your partner was tested for chlamydia, gonorrhea, syphilis, HIV, and hepatitis B. And although it's not routine for males, I'm also a fan of trichomoniasis testing for females. We will discuss herpes in question (e).

In addition, although the risk of sexual transmission is low, I recommend asking about recent hepatitis C testing if you're having sex with someone who uses IV drugs.

d. Were any of your tests positive?

In this chapter, we will focus on chlamydia, gonorrhea, hepatitis B, hepatitis C, herpes, HIV, HPV, syphilis, and trichomoniasis. But, of course, if they tested positive for any other STI, ask them what their doctor recommended in regard to sexual activity.

If your partner was treated for one of the following *and they didn't become reinfected after the treatment*, this is when it's safe for you to have sex with them:

- **Chlamydia.** If their doctor prescribed a medicine to take for seven days, they should wait until they've taken all the doses before having sex. If their doctor prescribed a single dose of medication, they should wait seven days after taking the medicine before having sex. You should also make sure all their symptoms have resolved because if they still have symptoms, that could mean they have another STI like trich, have been reinfected, or didn't take their medication properly.[5]
- **Gonorrhea.** They should wait seven days after treatment. As with chlamydia, you should make sure all their symptoms have resolved.[6]

- **Syphilis.** They should abstain from sexual contact until they're fully treated and their syphilis sores are completely healed. To be safe, ask them, "Did your doctor tell you that you can have sex?"[7]
- **Trichomoniasis.** Wait until they've been treated and all symptoms have gone away. This usually takes about a week.[8]

If they have one of the following viral infections, this is what I suggest:

- **Hepatitis B.** I recommend that you speak to your healthcare practitioner before having sex so that you can determine if you need a hepatitis B vaccine and so you understand your potential risks. Wear a latex condom to protect yourself.
- **Hepatitis C.** It's not common to transmit hepatitis C during sex, but it's possible. Treatment is available, but there is no vaccine for it. Talk to your doctor to make sure you understand the risks before having sex. Wear a latex condom to prevent transmission.
- **HIV.** I recommend abstaining from sex until you understand the risks and you've discussed pre-exposure prophylaxis (PrEP) with your doctor. PrEP reduces the risk of getting HIV from sex by about 99 percent when taken as prescribed.[9]

Genital herpes is discussed in the next question, and HPV is reviewed in question 12.

e. Have you ever been diagnosed with herpes simplex virus (HSV)?

Even when people are honest about other STDs, if they aren't having an active outbreak, they might not mention herpes. So after you ask about the other STIs, I recommend that you ask questions specifically about the herpes virus.

There are two types of herpes simplex virus (HSV): herpes simplex virus type 1 (HSV-1) and herpes simplex virus type 2 (HSV-2). HSV-1 usually causes sores on the lips or mouth (known as cold sores or fever blisters), but it can also cause genital infections too. HSV type 2 almost always causes genital sores, but it can occasionally infect the lips or mouth. Clinicians cannot tell the difference between the two types by physical examination alone, but a blood test or a swab of the lesion can differentiate between HSV-1 and HSV-2.

In the United States, about 1 out of every 6 people aged fourteen to forty-nine have genital herpes.[10] And approximately 50 percent of US adults have oral herpes.[11] If you have herpes at one site, it is rare to get the same type at another site. This is because once you are exposed to HSV-1 or HSV-2, your body makes antibodies to that particular type of HSV. For example, let's say you have HSV-1 antibodies because you had a cold sore in the past. Well, if someone with a cold sore that is also due to HSV-1 performs oral sex on you, it is not likely that you will get genital herpes, because your antibodies will prevent this from happening.

A person is more likely to transmit genital or oral herpes when a visible herpetic lesion is present, but it's still possible to transmit the virus if they don't have a sore. Even if your partner has no clue that they have genital herpes or a cold sore, they can still give it to you during vaginal, anal, or oral sex. Then you could end up having repeated outbreaks. Once you are infected, you will have the herpes simplex virus for the rest of your life.

Genital herpes caused by HSV-2 is much more likely to cause recurrent outbreaks. People with herpes can take a daily antiviral medication to prevent outbreaks and decrease the chance of spreading it to uninfected partners.

f. Do you have any STIs or STDs that I need to know about?

This is getting technical, but this will give them an opportunity to tell you about any known STIs/STDs they didn't mention before.

g. Do you have any ulcers, discharge/drips, or any other concerning symptoms that a doctor hasn't looked at yet?

If their answer to this question isn't a very confident no, that's a major red flag.

Note: People tend to love sex. A whole lot. So much so that a lot of them will lie to you about STI screening or STD status in order to have sex with you. So remember that even when you ask the right questions, not everyone is emotionally invested in your health or the health of your genitalia. What I'm saying is … when it comes to your sexual partners, choose wisely. If you and/or your partner is looking for somewhere to get tested in the United States, you can go to gettested.cdc.gov to find a testing center near you.

Question 8: Dr. Nita, that's a lot of questions to ask when I'm just trying to get some. Can I just skip that conversation and use a male condom (external condom) instead?

Nope. I don't recommend that. Not at all.

Some STIs, like chlamydia, gonorrhea, trichomoniasis, HIV, and hepatitis B are spread through sexual fluids, like semen. Condoms do a great job protecting you from those infections — assuming that the condom doesn't break or slip off, and assuming it is put on correctly before any sexual contact and it's the right size. (Hint: Not everyone needs an extra-large). But some STIs, such as herpes, HPV, and syphilis, are usually spread through skin-to-skin contact. That means that although condoms provide some protection when used correctly, you can still get herpes, HPV, or syphilis if your uncovered skin rubs against their infected uncovered skin, even if there is no penetration.

Wearing a condom and asking the questions we discussed is like wearing a seat belt even though you have an airbag in your car.

Note: Some STIs, including hepatitis B, hepatitis C, and HIV, are also spread through blood.

Question 9: Do some types of male (external) condoms work better than others?

Yes. Not all condoms provide the same level of protection. This is how I rate the options:

First place — latex condoms. In the world of condoms, latex is the g.o.a.t. (greatest of all time). We have the most studies supporting their effectiveness for both pregnancy and STI protection. If you and your partner(s) don't have a latex sensitivity or allergy, pick this one. But remember not to use oil-based lubricants or medications because they could weaken the condom and cause it to break. That means you should say no to items like cooking oil or whipped cream. Instead, use a silicone- or water-based lubricant. Tip: If you or your partner have an allergic reaction after exposure to latex condoms but not after exposure to other latex-containing products, the latex may not be the issue. You may be allergic or sensitive to brand-specific condom attributes, such as lubricants, perfumes, spermicides (chemicals that deactivate sperm), local anesthetics, or other chemical agents added during the manufacturing process. In this case, try switching to a different brand of latex condoms.

Second place — nonlatex condoms, which include plastic (polyurethane) or synthetic (polyisoprene) rubber condoms. If you can't use latex because of an allergy or sensitivity, one of these is your next-best option. We believe they're as effective as latex for protecting you from STIs, and they do a great job preventing pregnancy. You can use water-based or silicone lube with polyurethane and polyisoprene condoms. Oil-based products may also be safely used with polyurethane condoms. However, these types of condoms break more frequently than latex condoms.

A very distant third place — natural membrane (aka natural skin or lambskin) condoms. This type of condom has small pores that allow viruses like HIV and hepatitis B to pass through. So even though they can help prevent pregnancy, they should not be used for STI protection.

A few additional tips: Don't reuse external condoms. And whatever kind of condom you use, don't "double bag." Wearing two condoms increases the risk of breakage. Also, condoms should be stored in a cool dry place, and don't forget to always check the expiration date!

Question 10: Would I be better off using a female (internal) condom instead of a male (external) condom?

You can use an internal condom, but they aren't considered superior to male condoms. Although we *think* they provide similar protection from STIs, they haven't been studied nearly as much as male condoms. And if you are using them for pregnancy prevention, they actually have a higher failure rate. Twenty-one out of every hundred people get pregnant during the first year of using a female condom, compared to thirteen with a male condom. So if you do use a condom of the female variety for pregnancy prevention, you can consider adding another layer of protection like spermicidal foam, jelly, or cream. However, no type of spermicide (including those with nonoxynol-9, or N-9) will protect you from sexually transmitted infections (including HIV). Furthermore, spermicides may cause you to have a decreased number of good bacteria in your vagina, and they increase the risk of urinary tract infections for women.[12]

Plus, they're also pretty expensive ($3 to $7 each), and some women complain about crackling or popping noises that the condom makes during sex.[13]

A few additional tips: Don't reuse internal condoms. Don't use a male condom and a female condom at the same time. Friction between them can cause them to bunch up or tear. And make sure the penis doesn't insert on the side of the condom.

Question 11: What should I do to protect myself during oral sex?

You should always use a latex, polyurethane, or polyisoprene condom when performing oral sex on a penis and a dental dam when performing or receiving oral sex on the vulva, vagina, or anus. A dental dam is a sheet that creates a barrier between the mouth and the vagina or anus during oral sex. You can buy ready-to-use dental dams online or make your own using a latex, polyurethane, or polyisoprene condom. Just cut open a condom to make a square and put it between your mouth and your partner's genitals or anus (search the internet; they're easy to make). Alternatively, the FDA recently cleared ultrathin panties that can be worn to reduce the risk of STIs during oral sex. The single-use latex underwear, sold as Lorals for Protection, currently cost $25.00 for a pack of four.

Question 12: You haven't said much about the human papillomavirus (HPV). My friend told me that practically everyone gets it at some point in their life. Is that true? What do I need to know about it?

Your friend is right, which is why I wanted to give HPV its own section.

Genital HPV is the most common STI in the United States. By age fifty, at least 4 out of every 5 women will have been infected with HPV at some point in their lives.

The strains of HPV that infect the genital region and the mouth or throat can be separated into two main categories: low risk (wart causing) and high risk (precancer or cancer causing). In most cases the immune system clears or suppresses the virus within one to two years, before it causes any health problems. But if your immune system isn't able to defeat the virus, it can create health issues. Unfortunately, there is no way to predict who will clear the virus and who will go on to have warts, precancer, or cancer.

If your body isn't able to suppress a *low-risk* HPV infection, that can lead to anogenital warts (warts on the anus or genitals) or mouth/throat warts with oral sex. Testing for *low-risk* HPV isn't recommended. So people usually only know they have it if they have a history of warts.

If your body isn't able to suppress a *high-risk* HPV infection, that can lead to precancers and cancers of the cervix, vulva, vagina, or anus (or mouth and/or throat with oral sex). Women who are thirty or older usually get checked for high-risk HPV with their Pap smears. We typically only check for high-risk HPV in women who are under thirty if they have certain Pap smear abnormalities. (See chapter 11 for more details on Pap smears.) There is no FDA-approved test to screen men for high-risk HPV.

There is a vaccine for HPV that protects you against nine of the strains of the virus — some of which can cause cancer and some of which can cause warts. Since the vaccine will prevent you from getting HPV but won't cure any strains you already have, it's best to get it before you become sexually active. The recommended age to get it is eleven to twelve, but it's FDA approved for females and males aged nine to forty-five.[14]

It is important that women continue to be screened for cervical cancer, even after getting all recommended shots of the HPV vaccine. This is because the vaccine does not protect against *all* types of cervical cancer.

Question 13: My Pap smear has always been normal. Now HPV has popped up. Did my partner cheat on me?

A positive HPV test doesn't equal cheating. We're still learning about how the body handles this virus. We think some people may completely clear the virus, but others have it in a latent form, which means it's "hiding" in their cells so it doesn't show up on a Pap test for a while. But then it can become reactivated months or years later, suddenly showing up on the Pap.

So while your positive HPV test could be from a recent new exposure that might indicate that somebody cheated, it could also be from sex you had before you met your partner. Or perhaps it's just popping up on your Pap, but your partner gave it to you when you first started having sex with them.

Question 14: Is it possible to get an STI from a toilet seat?

It is highly unlikely.

Question 15: What are the treatments for the different STIs/STDs?

The following are the current recommendations for nonpregnant adults and adolescents without HIV who have genital infections. Recommendations are subject to change.

For individuals who have HIV but no other STD/STI,

antiretroviral therapy (ART) medication regimens will vary. Make sure your healthcare practitioner is knowledgeable about current ART recommendations.

Chlamydia

- **Recommended regimen.** Doxycycline 100 mg (milligrams) orally 2 times/day for 7 days
- **Alternative regimens.** Azithromycin 1 g orally in a single dose *or* levofloxacin 500 mg orally once daily for 7 days

Gonorrhea

- **Recommended regimen.** Ceftriaxone intramuscular shot in a single dose — 500 mg for people who weigh less than 330 pounds; 1 g for people weighing 330 pounds or more. *If chlamydial infection has not been ruled out, practitioners should also treat for chlamydia with doxycycline 100 mg orally 2 times a day for 7 days.*
- **Alternative regimens.**
  - For people allergic to the recommended medication: gentamicin 240 mg intramuscular in a single dose *plus* azithromycin 2 g orally in a single dose
  - If ceftriaxone administration is not available or not feasible: cefixime 800 mg orally in a single dose; if chlamydial infection has not been excluded, practitioners should treat for chlamydia with doxycycline 100 mg orally 2 times a day for 7 days.

Herpes

- **Recommended regimen for your first genital herpes outbreak.** *Treatment can be extended if healing is* *incomplete after 10 days of therapy.* Acyclovir 400 mg orally 3 times/day for 7–10 days (acyclovir 200 mg orally five times/day is also effective but is not recommended because of the frequency of dosing); *or* famciclovir 250 mg orally 3 times/day for 7–10 days; *or* valacyclovir 1,000 mg orally 2 times/day for 7–10 days

- **Recommended regimen for episodic genital herpes outbreak.** *Treatment is most effective if therapy is started within one day of getting a herpes lesion or during the prodrome (burning, pain, or itching) that comes before some outbreaks.* Acyclovir 800 mg orally 2 times/day for 5 days (acyclovir 400 mg orally 3 times/day is also effective, but is not recommended because of frequency of dosing); *or* acyclovir 800 mg orally 3 times/day for 2 days; *or* famciclovir 1 g orally 2 times/day for 1 day; *or* famciclovir 500 mg once, followed by 250 mg 2 times/day for 2 days; *or* famciclovir 125 mg 2 times/day for 5 days; *or* valacyclovir 500 mg orally 2 times/day for 3 days; *or* valacyclovir 1 g orally once daily for 5 days

- **Recommended regimen to prevent future genital herpes outbreak.** *This is for people who have frequent or severe outbreaks and/or those who want to decrease the risk of transmission to their HSV-uninfected sexual partner — regardless of symptom severity.* Acyclovir 400 mg orally 2 times/day; *or* valacyclovir 1 g orally once a day; *or* valacyclovir 500 mg orally once a day (note: valacyclovir 500 mg once a day might be less effective than other valacyclovir or acyclovir dosing regimens for persons who have frequent recurrences — i.e., 10 or more episodes/year); *or* famciclovir 250 mg orally 2 times/day

Low-risk HPV (genital warts)

- **Recommended treatments for external vulvar or anal warts.** *Optimal treatment option depends on size, number, location, and patient preference. If warts are not bothersome, treatment is not strictly necessary. Genital warts may go away on their own, but sometimes they get larger or grow in number. If you do opt for treatment, remember that you're removing the warts, but unless your body resolves the infection you'll still have the HPV that causes them. Therefore, some people will get warts again.*
  - **Patient-applied options.** Imiquimod cream, podophyllotoxin, or sinecatechins
  - **Healthcare practitioner–administered options.** Trichloroacetic acid (TCA) or bichloroacetic acid (BCA), cryotherapy (freezing), surgical removal (including laser removal or electrosurgery)
- **Recommended treatment options for vaginal warts** (healthcare practitioner–administered). TCA or BCA, cryotherapy, or surgical removal

High-risk HPV (precancers and cancers of cervix, vulva, or vagina)

- Treatment will vary depending on the severity of the lesion(s)

Syphilis, primary, secondary, and early latent (infection lasting less than one year)

- **Recommended regimen.** Benzathine penicillin G 2.4 million units intramuscular in a single dose
- **Alternative regimen.** Studies confirming the best treatments for penicillin-allergic patients are limited. Some options include doxycycline, tetracycline, and ceftriaxone.

Syphilis, late latent (infection lasting more than one year in duration)

- **Recommended regimen.** Benzathine penicillin G, administered as 3 intramuscular (IM) doses of 2.4 million units each, at 1-week intervals

Syphilis, tertiary with normal cerebrospinal fluid examination

- **Recommended regimen.** Benzathine penicillin G, 3 IM doses of 2.4 million units each, at 1-week intervals

Trichomoniasis

- **Recommended regimen for women.** Metronidazole 500 mg 2 times/day for 7 days
- **Recommended regimen for men.** Metronidazole 2 g orally in a single dose
- **Alternative regimens (same for women and men).** Tinidazole 2 g orally in a single dose

Question 16: What are some of the long-term consequences of untreated STDs?

In addition to the fact that STDs like chlamydia, gonorrhea, syphilis, herpes, trichomoniasis, and HIV can cause pregnancy complications or be passed from mom to baby during childbirth, here's the rundown of some other things that can happen if you aren't treated:

- **Chlamydia or gonorrhea.** Untreated chlamydia or gonorrhea can cause infertility, pelvic inflammatory disease (PID), and chronic pelvic pain, and they can increase your risk of an ectopic pregnancy. Occasionally, untreated gonorrhea can also spread to your blood or joints, and that can be life-threatening. Chlamydia may cause a reaction throughout the body known as reactive arthritis. This can lead to joint pain, pink eye, and/or a rash.

- **Genital herpes.** Open sores can make you more vulnerable to contracting HIV. Plus, a history of genital herpes can have an impact during pregnancy.[15] C-section is indicated in pregnant women with active genital herpes sores or symptoms such as vulvar pain or burning at delivery, because these symptoms may indicate viral shedding. And that would make it unsafe for the baby to pass through the birth canal. So if you have ever been diagnosed with genital herpes, be sure to tell your obstetrician. To help avoid the need for a C-section, when you are thirty-six weeks pregnant, they should start you on a medication (such as acyclovir) to help ensure that you are not having a genital herpes outbreak when it is time for you to deliver your baby.[16] And, of course, they will treat any outbreaks you have during pregnancy.

- **HIV.** For people living with HIV who are not diagnosed or taking ART, signs of HIV-related illness may develop within five to ten years, although it can be sooner. The time between HIV transmission and an AIDS diagnosis is usually ten to fifteen years, but it's sometimes longer. A very small number of people manage to control the HIV infection without ART and are called "elite-controllers." This situation is very rare. Most people will need ART to avoid becoming ill.

- **High-risk HPV.** If your HPV causes precancerous changes, catching it and treating it early can prevent progression to cancer.[17]

- **Syphilis.** There are four stages of syphilis: primary, secondary, latent, and tertiary. The symptoms you notice will depend on which stage you are in and what organ is infected. At any stage described below, syphilis can spread to the brain and nervous system (neurosyphilis), the eye (ocular syphilis), or the ear (otosyphilis).[18]

  ○ Primary stage: You might notice a single sore or multiple sores wherever the syphilis first entered your body. The sores, known as chancres, are usually round, firm, and painless. They typically last three to six weeks, and they heal even if you don't get treated. But even after the sore goes away, treatment is needed to prevent secondary syphilis.

  ○ Secondary stage: This stage typically starts with a rash on one or more areas of your body. This rash, which usually won't itch, can show up when your primary sore is still healing or several weeks after the sore has healed. Sometimes the rash is so faint that people miss it. Other things you may notice include patchy hair loss, fever, fatigue, or headache. The symptoms from this stage will go away whether or not you receive treatment. But without the right treatment, your infection will move to the latent and possibly tertiary stages of syphilis.

  ○ Latent stage: During this stage, which can last for years, there are no visible signs or symptoms of syphilis. Without treatment, you can continue to have syphilis in your body for years.

  ○ Tertiary stage: Most people with untreated syphilis do not develop tertiary syphilis. However, when it does happen, it can affect many different organ systems, including the brain, heart, and nervous system. Tertiary syphilis, which can result in death, would occur ten to thirty years after the initial infection.[19]

Question 17: What should I do if I get a sexually transmitted infection or disease?

First of all, know that it's OK to have a lot of feelings and questions when you're diagnosed with an STI or STD. But no matter how you're feeling, remember that your diagnosis doesn't define you, and you're not alone. Over half of Americans will get an STI at some point in their lifetimes. Don't hesitate to ask your doctor questions. It's their job to treat you, and you should never feel judged. If you do, get a new doctor!

Make sure you understand your treatment plan, and ask if you need to be retested or have a follow-up exam. For example, women should be retested three months after finishing treatment for chlamydia, gonorrhea, or trichomoniasis.[20] You also need to make sure all your recent sexual partners are notified.

Question 18: Dr. Nita, you say to notify all my recent partners if I find out I have an STI, but how do I approach this subject?

It's important to tell your partner(s) about any STIs you are diagnosed with. Otherwise, you could put their health at risk, as well as the health of anyone else they have sex with. Here are some things to consider:

- If you're afraid to tell your partner, your doctor (or the person who diagnosed your STI) may be willing to contact them for you and not disclose your information. Or your local health department might be able to help you with partner notification. Alternatively, if you go to online services such as STDcheck.com or tel-lyourpartner.org, you can enter your partner's phone number or email and they will receive an anonymous text about the exposure.

- If you're concerned that your partner will become angry, please don't disclose your diagnosis in a confined space that might be unsafe if your partner reacts in a violent manner. Instead, use one of the services listed above, text them, or meet them in a safe public place but one where you can have a private conversation. If you're meeting them in person and you're nervous, plan ahead what you're going to say. Be open and honest, and prepare yourself for their questions. Then give them time to process the news if they need it.

- Try to avoid getting defensive, and stay calm, even if they get upset.

- If the conversation remains civil, see if you can find out if they have a history of STIs/STDs.[21] Remember, though, that you might have actually gotten the STI from the person you're talking to.

Your New Normal (If It Isn't Already Your Normal)

I know the info in this chapter is a lot to take in, and some of it is scary. But one of the reasons STDs are so common is that we aren't having the conversations about them that we need to have. We should live in a world where it's the norm to have a fun, satisfying sexual relationship while still staying safe. So ask questions. And if something inside tells you it isn't a good idea to have sex with someone — sit that sex session *out*. Don't play Russian roulette with your health.

Part II

COMMON WOMEN'S HEALTH ISSUES

Advocate for Your Health Like a Pro

Chapter 6

Finding Dr. Right

Tips for Finding a Doctor You Actually Like

I was a medical student on an obstetrics and gynecology rotation, and it had been a hell of a week (in a good way). On Monday we told "Ms. June," a seventy-year-old patient who'd been battling recurrent cancer, that her scans were clear. She threw her hands up as she shouted, "Thank you, Jesus!" Then, she jumped out of her chair, pulled a portable radio out of her purse, turned it up as loud as it would go, and did a dance the likes of which I'd never seen before (or since). Her happiness was so contagious that within two minutes, everybody in the room was dancing with her.

On Tuesday I watched a thirty-five-year-old stroke patient take her first steps in rehab. Her husband, who had been by her side the entire time, could barely contain himself. I had never seen a man cry so many tears of joy.

On Thursday we told three women who had been struggling with infertility that they were pregnant. Not one, not two, but *three* women!

That Friday morning, I was on top of the world as I sang and danced to Beyoncé while driving to the hospital. I thought to myself, "This is why I want to become a doctor: healing and happiness." Once I parked, I hopped out of my car, headed into the hospital, and logged in to complete my first task: checking daily labs and pathology reports. I typed in the information for the first patient: "B-r-e-n-d-a." But when I saw her results, I thought, "Wait… that can't be right. Her biopsy came back as cancerous?"

Based on Brenda's age, family history, and symptoms, the surgeon was almost certain her results would be benign. It was immediately clear to me that Friday wasn't going to be a good day, and it wasn't. The doctor in charge was compassionate and supportive when she broke the news. But Brenda, who was a single mom with three kids and no support system, was understandably terrified.

There was no singing or dancing on the way home that Friday night. Instead, I ugly cried for Brenda, for her children, and for all the women in similar situations. By the time I got home, I was an emotional wreck. As I walked into my house with mascara running down my face, I decided I'd made a huge career mistake. After thinking about it for a few hours, I came up with the perfect solution. I decided to quit medicine.

But by Sunday, after doing some research, learning more about the effective treatment options Brenda could choose from, and finding different financial programs that could help her, I felt better and decided to unquit medicine.

That Monday morning, I showed up to the hospital bright-eyed and bushy-tailed, but by Friday afternoon, my bright eyes were once again red and puffy from ugly crying. And my tail was no longer bushy. I'd been present for five cancer diagnoses and three miscarriage diagnoses. Plus, my attending (the doctor in charge) had tasked me with telling a married woman that her husband had given her a sexually transmitted infection called trichomoniasis.

After delivering all that bad news and watching patients' reactions that ranged from anger to denial to confusion, I felt as if my mind, body, and soul had just lost a fight with the heavyweight champion of the world. And I wanted to quit medicine ... again.

But then, as I was leaving the hospital that night, I heard someone yelling my name. When I turned around, it was Mr. Benton, a cardiac patient I'd cared for when I was working with the internal medicine team. The doctors didn't think he'd leave the hospital alive, but there he was, living and breathing. Going home. I sat and chatted with him while he waited for his son to pull the car around. His eyes were full of joy as he told me how he couldn't wait to sit on the couch with his wife and watch cowboy movies while playing with his new grand-baby. When his son arrived, the nurse helped him get into the car, and we said goodbye. Right before they pulled off, he rolled down the window and shouted, "I hope I never see y'all again," then he waved at us and chuckled as they drove away.

Talking to Mr. Benton was like seeing a beautiful rainbow after a horrible storm. As I drove home from the hospital that night, I realized I was looking at the situation all wrong. Yes, crappy, unfair stuff happens to patients in doctors' offices and hospitals every day. But not all trials end in tragedy. Some end in triumph. Thousands of cancer patients turn into cancer sur-vivors. Thanks to advancements in fertility treatments, there are miracle babies running around on playgrounds all around the world. And some people have recovery stories that are so miraculous that when doctors are asked how it happened, they can't do anything but shrug their shoulders and scratch their heads.

As I thought about it, I realized that some of the unex-pected patient trials from my very bad week would turn into testimonies that would give hope to others in similar situations.

And for patients who didn't get the outcomes they were hoping and praying for, I could be a source of knowledge and encouragement.

By the time I got home, I felt empowered. I realized that my patients didn't need a doctor who curled up into a ball every time bad news was delivered. They needed and deserved someone who would stand up and help them reclaim control of their lives when an unexpected trial popped up. So instead of quitting medicine, I decided to do the opposite. I decided to become the best damn doctor I could be.

That day, I set out to answer one of the most important questions I ever asked myself during my med school training: "When life takes a swing at a patient, what is the best way for a doctor to help them fight back?"

Of course, having the medical knowledge and skills to take care of a patient is a given. But I felt that an important emotional aspect to patient care was being ignored. So I came up with a plan to figure out how to bridge that emotional gap.

Part of every medical student's education is called "rounds." This is how rounding typically worked for rotations. Every morning at a ridiculously early time, medical students would arrive at the hospital first to see all the patients on the service. Then, later that morning, the attending would come in to oversee everything, quizzing us and explaining how to do procedures. We also went to each patient's room together to watch the attendings as they interacted with the patients we'd seen earlier that morning. We would get to hear what additional questions the attendings asked, how they performed the physical exam, what treatments they recommended, and so on.

There were several attending physicians on my rotation. So if a patient was in the hospital for a while, I had an opportunity to watch different attendings interact with them. I knew the patients always got great care because all my attendings were incredibly knowledgeable, but they all had very different styles. During the course of my rotation, these are the different types I discovered:

- **The Explainer.** All attendings make sure their patients understand what's most important, but this doctor took explaining to the next level. The doc was known for printing articles for the patient that reviewed everything from how their medical condition was discovered to the evolution of diagnostic capabilities and possible future treatment options.
- **The Bonder.** This doctor would sit and listen to patients talk about everything. If the patient's dog had five puppies, she would know all their names.
- **The Prayer.** While she never forced her beliefs on anyone, if a patient mentioned they were religious, she would happily pray with them every day.
- **The Give It to 'Em Straight Doctor.** This very matter-of-fact attending showed absolutely no emotion while interacting with patients. This doc believed his way was the right way. Period.
- **The Holistic Healer.** They believed that complete healing only happened if a person's mind, body, and spirit were properly cared for.
- **The Cheerleader.** This attending acknowledged what was going wrong with a patient's health but also highlighted what was going right. She loved celebrating patient wins, both big and small. If a patient lost five pounds, she would damn near break out a tuba and start playing a celebratory song.

For my social experiment, I wanted to observe how each patient responded to these very different personalities. Was one physician personality superior to another in gaining a patient's trust and compliance? Who would patients respond to the best?

I didn't know it at the time, but a patient we will call "Mrs. Hannah" turned out to be the perfect person to kick off my study. Day one of my experiment was day four of her hospitalization.

Mrs. Hannah was a feisty seventy-five-year-old African American woman who was constantly in and out of the hospital for various medical issues. It was a never-ending cycle: she would be admitted to the hospital, doctors would come up with a treatment plan, she would be discharged, and she'd soon be readmitted because of a flare-up due to her noncompliance with the plan.

During this hospitalization, I had an opportunity to get to know Mrs. H. pretty well. Every morning when I went to examine her, she'd smile and say, "Hey, baby." Then in the midst of answering my questions and allowing me to perform my daily physical exam, she would give me a list of chores. She'd ask me to get her a blanket, grab her some ice, turn on the TV, and so on.

Each day, as I was completing the random tasks on her to-do list, we would chitchat about different things. On this particular day, she started telling me about one of her family members who had taken part in the Tuskegee experiment. In case you're not familiar with that atrocity, in 1932 the United States Public Health Service started a program called the Tuskegee Study of Untreated Syphilis in the Negro Male. It initially involved six hundred impoverished Black men — 399 with syphilis and 201 who did not have the disease. The researchers told the men that they were receiving free medical care for "bad blood," a local term used to describe several illnesses. And to sweeten the deal, the researchers threw in some free meals and burial insurance. But none of the men (most of whom were illiterate) were told they had syphilis. Then, for forty years, the government's medical experiment allowed hundreds of African American men with syphilis to go untreated so that scientists could study the debilitating, deadly effects of the disease, even after penicillin was discovered as a cure in the 1940s. The men had no clue that they were being used as human guinea pigs while an effective treatment option was being withheld from them. The US government and participating local physicians stood by and watched these men die unnecessarily. They also did nothing as the men passed the deadly (but treatable) disease to their wives, some of whom passed it on to their unborn children during pregnancy.

After Mrs. Hannah finished the story, she said, "You can't trust what people tell you in here."

That was it! The doctors and social workers assumed she was noncompliant because of social issues, but the real reason was that she didn't trust doctors. And why should she? As I thought about her previous encounters with attendings, it all made sense. On day one of her hospitalization, the Explainer spent thirty minutes going over different studies and research options. When I walked in the room the next morning, those papers were in exactly the same place my attending had left them. Mrs. H. hadn't touched them because she didn't trust the information.

On day two, Mrs. H pretty much looked out the window the whole time the Give It to 'Em Straight Doctor was talking. She probably found him condescending and annoying.

On day three, she seemed less than impressed by the Holistic Healer, which makes sense. If she wasn't willing to let a doctor heal her body, there was no way she was going to let them near her mind or her spirit.

The day I figured out the root of the issue, the Bonder was rounding. That was perfect. After I told her that the patient had lost her faith in medical professionals, she knew exactly what to do.

When we got to the patient's room, the Bonder didn't just blurt out, "I heard you don't trust doctors." Instead, she sat down and had an authentic conversation with the patient that somehow led to Mrs. H. sharing her Tuskegee experiment story with us. By the end of the conversation, Mrs. H's body language had totally changed. I won't say that she was 100 percent ready to put her life in the hands of doctors, but we'd definitely made a lot of progress. For the first time during that hospitalization, she was at least willing to consider the treatment recommendations. That was one point for the Bonder. But as wonderful as she was, the Bonder wasn't everyone's preference.

For example, another patient named Rebecca, who loved yoga and meditated every day, valued the Holistic Healer's approach. Ms. Butler, a young CEO from New York, didn't want to bond with anyone and didn't feel the need to heal her spirit. She just wanted a Give It to 'Em Straight Doctor to tell her what was wrong and how to fix it. On the other hand, when Mrs. Johnson whipped out her long list of questions during rounds, the Explainer and her piles of research were a match made in heaven. The Cheerleader was like light in a very dark place for the teenage patient battling a sickle cell anemia crisis. And the Prayer was exactly what the doctor ordered for a patient named Lori, whose answer to every health obstacle was, "It'll be OK. God is good."

Over the next several months, I started playing doctor-patient matchmaker in outpatient clinics. I'd intentionally schedule patient follow-up appointments on the days the appropriately matched attendings would be working. Then I'd step back and enjoy the magic. Even when their treatment recommendations didn't change, I watched lots of noncompliant diabetics become compliant, I saw obese people shed pounds at an accelerated rate, and I listened to patients say yes to treatment options they'd previously refused. All because they liked the way the treatment plans were presented to them. All because they found their Dr. Right.

How to Find Your Dr. Right for Women's Health

Just like Mrs. Hannah and all the other patients I encountered, if you don't vibe with your doc for any reason, you might consciously or subconsciously put up a wall of distrust, and your health could suffer unnecessarily. If you truly want to be the healthiest version of yourself, you need to see doctors who make you feel respected, heard, and understood. Here are some tips for finding *your* Dr. Right. (I realize that some patients receive wonderful care from mid-level health professionals like nurse practitioners and midwives instead of doctors. These tips apply to them too!)

Know what type of doctor personality you want

You might desire different personality types in different types of doctors. For instance, for your primary care physician, who will help you manage health issues like diabetes and high blood pressure, maybe you'd like a cheerleader. But when it comes to your gynecologist, maybe you'd prefer an explainer. As long as the doctor is ethical and knowledgeable and has a solid skill set, there isn't a right or wrong personality preference.

Commit to taking your search seriously

Some people put as much thought into picking their women's health practitioner as they do into picking out fruit at the grocery store. That's a mistake because when you go to a doctor, you're trusting them with an invaluable asset: your health.

Plus, in addition to your immediate women's healthcare needs, there's another important perk of having a Dr. Right. If you get an unexpected diagnosis like cancer, or you need to be referred to another type of doctor, your trusted gynecologist — who knows lots of other doctors and who understands and respects your physician personality and treatment preferences — can tell you who would be a great match for you. Or if you're in a situation where you don't have many options because not a lot of doctors work in the field you need to be referred to, or your insurance limits your options, you might feel more confident in the care you're receiving if your trusted Dr. Right says something like, "You probably won't mesh well with this doctor, but trust me: they're phenomenal."

Ask your family, friends, and coworkers for recommendations

Sure, you can look on the internet or ask random strangers at the grocery store or beauty salon for recommendations, but since those people don't know you and you don't know them, you could be polar opposites when it comes to your physician personality preferences or needs. So their Dr. Right could be your Dr. Wrong.

If you want to improve your odds of finding your Dr. Right, focus on referrals from family and friends who have personalities and wants similar to yours. But even if your friends and family wouldn't pick the same doctor as you, at least they'd have a better idea of what type of doctor you might mesh with.

When you request recommendations, ask questions like, "Why do you like this doctor? Does she listen to your questions? Does she usually recommend conventional treatment options, or does she like to include lots of alternatives like herbal supplements?" If you're looking for a practitioner who's into holistic healing, you probably won't click with a gynecologist who doesn't believe that acupuncture or yoga can be beneficial.

Getting recommendations from coworkers with the same insurance plan is also a great idea... which brings me to my next tip.

Check with your insurance company

Nobody wants a surprise medical bill. So check with your insurance company to make sure the doctor you want to see is in their network. In-network doctors are contracted with your health plan to provide services for you usually at a lower cost than noncontracted doctors. If you choose to schedule an appointment with an out-of-network (noncontracted) doctor, you might end up paying a lot more.

Also, remember that although a doctor's clinic may be in-network, the hospital where the doctor has privileges may *not* be. That's why it's a good idea to find out which hospital(s) your physician works at. Then ask your insurance company if care at that hospital is covered by your plan. Even if you aren't expecting to be admitted to the hospital, it's nice to know if you'll have access to your doctor if you ever need to be hospitalized.

While you have your insurance company on the phone,

make sure you also understand all the fees and copays associated with your plan, and if there are different insurance plan tiers, ask about the pros and cons of each option.

Do some doctor research

Once you've decided on your Dr. Right contender(s), check out their credentials. An internet search can tell you if a doctor is licensed to practice, if they're board-certified or board-eligible, and whether they've had disciplinary action taken against them. An action doesn't always confirm something negative about a doctor, but if you see a repetitive pattern, that could suggest a problem.

Go on your doctor date

Now it's time to see if the doctor-patient relationship is going to work out. But before you go, keep these three tips in mind. First, even if you've seen a string of Dr. Not So Rights in the past, be willing to give your new doctor a chance to prove herself. Second, don't ignore your intuition, but don't have unrealistic expectations either. Doctors aren't magicians. Sometimes healing and treatment plans take time. You might need to have labs drawn or imaging tests ordered, or your doc might need to try out different treatment options to determine what works best for you. So even if a doctor is knowledgeable and a perfect personality match for you, it might take some time to figure out your diagnosis or determine your best treatment plan. And, last but not least, remember that the doctor is the leader of the team, but they're a package deal — they come with their staff. So if you don't enjoy interacting with the schedulers or nurses, or if you don't love the overall vibe of the office, take that into consideration as well.

DR. NITA'S NOTE
Ask Your Gynecologist If You Need a Primary Care Doctor

Some gynecologists consider themselves primary care doctors, and some internal medicine doctors and family practice doctors feel comfortable handling basic gynecological care like Pap smears and breast exams. But don't assume that your gynecologist is completing all the tasks that a primary care doctor would typically do or that your family practice or internal medicine physician is performing all the duties a gynecologist would usually undertake. If you want one doctor to serve as your primary care doctor and perform the duties of a gynecologist, make sure you ask them if they're OK with that plan. Otherwise, you might unknowingly neglect important aspects of your health, like fertility discussions, contraceptive counseling, or routine screenings to check for medical issues such as diabetes and high cholesterol.

If at first you don't succeed, try, try again

I understand and respect the fact that nobody has the time or desire to go on an excessive number of "doctor dates." But I also understand the potential harms of mismatched doctor-patient personalities. So don't give up. If possible, consider traveling a little farther from home if you aren't able to find your Dr. Right locally. Or, if your insurance company will pay for a telemedicine appointment, you might be able to be evaluated by a doctor who lives too far away for an in-person visit. (Telemedicine may not be the best option if your issue requires a physical exam, but even then, the clinician may be able to review your records to give you suggestions.) Remember to check in with your insurance company to find out how much your copay will be if you decide to try a few doctors out.

Once you've found your Dr. Right, he or she will make your visit to the doctor's office or hospital as pleasant as an appointment can be. You'll feel comfortable telling them anything they need to know to address your health, and you'll feel confident that they're giving you good advice. The relationship will feel easy and natural. Like your Dr. Right was created specifically for you.

But while you are searching for a better fit, don't ditch your Dr. Wrong before finding a new doc unless you have a very compelling reason for doing so — especially if you have on-going medical problems. That way, you'll have access to things like medication refills.

DR. NITA'S NOTE
Black Women's Health Spotlight

Blatant racism is hard to defend. *Most* individuals now agree that forcing people onto slave ships, stripping them of their names and culture, and treating them like trash while they worked for free in horrific conditions...was wrong. Burning crosses on people's front lawns and claiming that the color of your skin somehow magically makes you superior...is wrong. And using the N-word in an effort to make others feel inferior...is wrong. However, while practices such as those are typically no longer openly defended, less conspicuous, more socially palatable spin-offs of those examples — such as structural racism and implicit bias (we will define those later in this section) — have found an impressive number of ways to infiltrate almost every aspect of the Black American experience, including the healthcare field.

For example, Black newborn babies die at three times the rate of white newborns in the United States.[1] Additionally, compared to white women, Black women in the United States are three to four times as likely to die from pregnancy-related complications.[2] And, to be clear, no level of education and no amount of money in the bank makes Black families exempt from healthcare inequalities such as those. For instance, in one study, financially stable and college-educated Black women in New York City were more likely to experience severe maternal morbidity than white women who lived in poverty as well as white women without a high school diploma.[3] Of course, I'm not insinuating that money, education, status, or any other factor makes one life more valuable than another, but I don't want anyone reading this to think that having degrees or a lot of money makes them immune to this harsh reality.

For obvious reasons, I'm emotionally invested in the health of Black women. But a good doctor practices medicine based on facts, not emotions. So let's take my feelings out of the equation. What do respected experts and research studies say?

"Past work by a range of scholars has shown that 200 black people die every single day in these United States who would not have died if the health experience of African Americans was equivalent to that of whites." — 2020 statement from a Harvard University social scientist[4]

"Medical doctors, like the entire sample, showed an implicit preference for White Americans relative to Black Americans.... African American MDs, on average, did not show an implicit preference for either Blacks or Whites, and women showed less implicit bias than men." — *Journal of Health Care for the Poor and Underserved*[5]

"To be clear, structural racism exists in the U.S. and in medicine, genuinely affecting the health of all people, especially people of color and others historically marginalized in society. This is not opinion or conjecture, it is proven in numerous studies, through the science and in the evidence. As physicians, and as leaders in medicine, we have a responsibility to not only acknowledge and understand the impact of structural racism on the lives of our patients, but to speak out against racial injustices wherever they exist in health care and society." — 2021 statement from the American Medical Association[6]

Solid research doesn't lie. So in addition to the other info in this chapter, here are four tips to help you protect your health and the health of your loved ones.

1. **Watch out for structural racism.** *Structural racism* refers to the laws, rules, and practices in society that give preferential treatment and opportunities to one race over others. In medicine it shows up in obvious ways like healthcare facilities in predominantly Black neighborhoods that don't have access to cutting-edge technology or government policies that make it unnecessarily difficult for Black people to access healthcare. But it also shows up in more insidious ways. For instance, most patients don't realize that race is incorporated into a lot of medical decision-making formulas and tools that clinicians use to decide which treatment is right for you when it comes to a range of conditions. Even though we don't always have adequate scientific research to support the assumption that race matters, being Black frequently puts patients at a disadvantage when it comes to treatment for important medical matters. This may direct more attention and resources to white patients.[7] For more information about medical treatments that take race into account, read the article entitled "Hidden in

Plain Sight — Reconsidering the Use of Race Correction in Clinical Algorithms," which can be found at https://www .nejm.org/doi/full/10.1056/NEJMms2004740. (Of note, clinical algorithms are periodically updated. Your clinician can tell you if a particular algorithm still takes race into account.)

Even if your doctor is willing to walk through hell and high water to provide equal care for you, it's impossible to treat all patients equally when operating in a healthcare system that is inherently racist.

2. **Be mindful of implicit bias.** Based on my experience as a patient who has put her life in the hands of doctors who are not Black and as a physician who has worked side-by-side with physicians of all ethnicities, I feel 100 percent comfortable saying that the vast majority of physicians I've worked with aren't explicitly racist. However, when we put on our white coats, our life experiences and character flaws don't magically disappear. So something called *implicit bias*, which is unconscious favoritism toward or prejudice against a certain group of people, can come into play. Implicit bias occurs automatically and unintentionally, so your doctor won't realize that they are treating you differently.

3. Be aware that structural racism and implicit bias exist in medicine, but **don't assume that a doctor doesn't have your best interests at heart just because they don't look like you.** Just like I know incredible Black doctors, I also know equally incredible doctors who are not Black. To deprive yourself of either experience would be a mistake.

4. **Be open to the possibility that you could be talking to your Dr. Right.** Some patients have had so many negative experiences, they are understandably guarded when they see a new doctor. But try not to use your previous experiences in judging your current doctor.

Racism in medicine is a public health emergency, and the medical community hasn't done enough to right this wrong. Black, Indigenous, and other marginalized people of color deserve better.

Be a great patient

There's no way your doctor can do their best work without help from you. So when you show up for your appointment, be ready and willing to give your doctor all the information they need to help you on your healthcare journey. And remember that there's no need to lie. Don't say you work out three times a week if you haven't exercised in six months. And don't bend the truth about how long it's been since you had sex or how many sexual partners you've had. Think about it: if you tell your doctor about a hypothetical version of yourself who exercises three times a week, has been abstinent for seven years, and has only six ounces of wine every other New Year's Eve, your doctor will tell you which tests and screenings the hypothetical version of you should get. That doesn't do the real you any good! Frankly, it's a waste of your time and money, and it's a missed opportunity for you to get the care you need and deserve.

And once you have a treatment plan, be ready to do the work. If you don't implement your doctor's recommendations at home, your health won't reap the benefits.

Don't be afraid to switch it up

People grow and change, so your healthcare wants and needs may change. If your Dr. Right evolves into a Dr. Not So Right for You, start searching for another physician.

DR. NITA'S NOTE

Advocate for Your Health Like a Pro When Things Aren't Going Great

When you go to the doctor with a complaint that doesn't have a definite diagnosis, as your doctor is listening to you talk they're mentally putting the pieces of your story together to come up with a list of the possible reasons for your symptoms. That list of possibilities is called a "differential diagnosis." Or if they know what your diagnosis is, they are figuring out the best next steps.

Whichever scenario you're dealing with, you need to know what your doctor is thinking. So if you find yourself in a situation where your appointment is coming to an end but you have no clue what's going on in your doc's head, here's what I recommend:

Scenario 1: You Don't Have a Diagnosis Yet, and You Have No Clue What Your Doctor Thinks It Might Be

The best option is to say, "I didn't quite follow what happened during my appointment. Can you tell me … (fill in the blank with all your questions)?"

Here's the next-best option:

- Ask, "What are the top three things that might be causing what's going on with me?" In a lot of cases, the list of possible causes will include a lot more than three possibilities. However, asking for three will allow you to get a better sense of what's at the top of their list. (If your diagnosis is so textbook that they know what it is, they might give you only one answer.)

- If you don't write down their answer yourself or you aren't sure how to spell what the doctor is saying, your next question should be, "Can you or your nurse write that down for me?" It's tough for someone to say, "No, I won't tell you what I think you might have." Now you have something in writing in case you want to research it. Plus, if you see another doctor for the same complaint, you can see if their differential diagnoses match up. (Warning: As doctors, our minds frequently go to a dark place first because we don't want to miss anything that can harm you. So cancer pops up a lot in our differential diagnosis. It doesn't mean you definitely have cancer!)

- "Were you able to rule out anything important during today's evaluation? If so, what?" This will allow you to stay in the know when it comes to what they've already ruled out.

- If you're getting a list of labs or imaging, you can ask what the labs or the imaging will rule out.

If you see this doctor more than once, you can ask these questions at each visit until you have a diagnosis

Scenario 2: You Have a Diagnosis, but You Don't Understand the Next Steps

Say, "I don't understand the next steps. Can you repeat them and tell me why you think they're needed?" Then, once they tell you what they are, repeat the steps back as you understand them and end with, "Did I get that right?"

Whatever you do, please don't walk away with no idea of what happened. Even if your visit wasn't as pleasant as you'd like, and even if you are 100 percent sure you are going to get a second opinion on everything the doctor recommended, there's no harm in hearing what this doctor has to say.

The Game Plan

If you're one of the millions of women who are still searching for their Dr. Right, and you're sick and tired of walking away from appointments with more questions than answers, or if you want to get the most out of your visit with your Dr. Right, the rest of the chapters in this part of the book are for you.

This is not a comprehensive women's health brain dump. And since every woman is unique and no two doctors practice medicine exactly the same, the info in these chapters is not one-size-fits-all medical advice that can take the place of a doctor's visit, but if you walk into your doctor's appointment knowing what I'm about to tell you, you'll be prepped and primed to "patient like a pro," which I define as having the information you need to advocate for your health and get the answers you need and deserve.

Chapter 7

Let's Talk about Your Mood, Sis

PMS and PMDD

People laugh and joke about premenstrual syndrome (PMS) and premenstrual dysphoric disorder (PMDD), but what's the funny part? Is the joke …

Knock, knock.
Who's there?
A thirty-seven-year-old.
A thirty-seven-year-old who?
A thirty-seven-year-old who just yelled at her loving husband for forty-five minutes because he accidentally put the dishwasher on the pots and pans cycle instead of the regular cycle. Now she can't stop crying because she feels a deep emotional connection with a cute cat on Instagram who's struggling to jump onto the couch, and she simply can't understand why everybody in the comments is laughing instead of rooting for the cat.

Or maybe it's …

A twenty-seven-year-old who took sick days from work *again* because her PMS has sucked the energy out of her and left her with a headache, the acne of a fourteen-year-old, the joint pain of a senior citizen, and a level of bloating that can't be described in words.

Feel free to create your own scenario with any of the more than 150 symptoms associated with PMS/PMDD. No matter how you spin it, none of them are funny or fun for the person experiencing them (or the people around the person who's experiencing them). Feeling crappy or losing sick days to cramps, depression, or pounding headaches sucks. But as women, a lot of us have just learned to live with PMSing.

I want better for us.

Think about it. On average, women get their periods for about forty years of their lives. If a woman has PMS for one week a month, twelve months a year for forty years, that's 3,360 days of PMS suffering. I don't want you to power through that. I want you to understand what's going on, and I want you to know what you can do about it.

PMS/PMDD CRASH COURSE
What You Need to Know to Patient Like a Pro

Question 1: Why am I like this?

Question 2: Can PMS or PMDD be diagnosed with a physical exam or a blood test?

Question 3: How do I find out if I have PMS or PMDD?

Question 4: Can I still have PMS or PMDD if I don't have a period every month?

Question 5: If I have it, at what age will it pop up, and when will it go away?

Question 6: I don't want to take hormones to treat my symptoms. But this PMS has got to go. What can I do?

Question 7: I'm going to need more than a nap and some vitamins. PMS/PMDD is about to have me single (or maybe
even fired or in jail if my coworker doesn't back off). If my
main problem is my mood, what else can I do?

Question 8: If physical symptoms are my main complaint, or
if my mood symptoms don't go away with SSRIs, what
do you recommend?

Question 9: What if none of those suggestions work?

Question 10: How long will I need to take meds to control my
PMS/PMDD symptoms?

Let's look at these questions one at a time.

Question 1: Why am I like this?

No one knows for sure what causes PMS or PMDD symptoms,
but here's what we think happens. If you don't get pregnant
after ovulation (which is when your ovary releases an egg to
be fertilized by a sperm), your estrogen and progesterone levels start falling dramatically (figure 6). When those hormones
take a nose-dive, PMS/PMDD symptoms begin. Then, PMS/
PMDD symptoms go away within a few days after a woman's
period starts as hormone levels begin rising again.

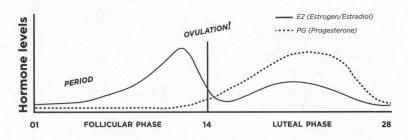

Figure 6. Hormone changes in an average cycle

Note: Women with PMS and PMDD have the same amount of estrogen and progesterone as women who don't have these conditions. However, for unknown reasons, people with PMS/PMDD seem to be more sensitive to the normal changes in hormone levels that happen during menstrual cycles.

In addition to playing a role when it comes to the physical symptoms associated with PMS and PMDD, rising and falling levels of estrogen and progesterone may also have an impact on chemicals in the brain — including one called serotonin. Basically, people with PMS/PMDD don't have enough serotonin after ovulation, and that may contribute to issues like food cravings, premenstrual depression, sleep problems, fatigue, and other symptoms that suck the joy out of life.

Common PMS/PMDD symptoms include the following:

Abdominal pain or cramps
Acne flare-ups
Anger or aggression
Anxiety
Arguments with people
Backache
Binge eating
Bloating or swelling
Breast tenderness or
    swelling
Constipation
Crying spells
Decreased interest in
    usual activities
Decreased productivity at
    home, work, or school
Depressed or sad mood
Diarrhea
Difficulty concentrating

Distractedness
Dizziness
Fatigue
Feeling overwhelmed
Food cravings
Forgetfulness
Headache
Hot flashes
Irritability
Joint or muscle pain or
    stiffness
Low sexual desire
Mood swings
Oily skin
Overeating
Oversensitivity
Sleeping too much
Trouble falling asleep
Weight gain

Question 2: Can PMS or PMDD be diagnosed with a physical exam or a blood test?

No. There are no unique physical exam findings or lab tests that can confirm or rule out a diagnosis of PMS or PMDD. However, your doctor might order labs to check for other problems that can mimic PMS/PMDD (e.g., thyroid issues).

Question 3: How do I find out if I have PMS or PMDD?

The diagnosis is based on your symptoms. Let's start by talking about a PMS diagnosis.

PMS Diagnostic Quiz

If you answer yes to all three of these questions, you may have PMS. If you answer no to any of the questions, you do not have PMS.

	Yes	No
1. Have you had physical or behavioral symptoms that were present in the five days before your period started for at least two menstrual cycles in a row?	❏	❏
2. Did your symptoms *totally disappear* by the fourth day of your period?	❏	❏
3. Did your symptoms keep you from enjoying or doing some of your normal activities (like school, work, or social events)?	❏	❏

Questions 1 and 2 are important because people with PMS only experience symptoms between ovulation and the first few days of their period. Once their hormone levels increase, their physical and emotional symptoms disappear. Question 3 matters because if your symptoms aren't bothersome enough to keep you from enjoying or doing some of your normal activities, you don't meet the criteria for a PMS diagnosis.

Now let's discuss PMDD.

The timing of PMDD symptoms is the same as it is for PMS: they are present during the week before a person's period and improve once the period starts. But when it comes to severity of symptoms, PMDD is like PMS on steroids (especially for emotional symptoms such as mood swings, anger, irritability, internal tension, anxiety, depression, and increased sensitivity to rejection). Going into detail about the specific criteria used to diagnose a person with PMDD goes beyond the scope of this book, but if your mood symptoms are particularly intense and you think you might have PMDD, schedule an appointment with a clinician to get evaluated. Hint: A lot of patients (and their partners) think they have PMDD, but they don't. PMDD impacts only about 2 to 5 percent of reproductive-age women.

If you want to track your symptoms to determine if you have PMS or PMDD, there are lots of great apps you can use, or you can google "free printable PMS symptom tracker" to get a list of free charts you can use. You can refer to the list of common symptoms on page 138 as a guide, but remember that there are over 150 psychological, behavioral, and physical symptoms. If you have a symptom that is not on the list, still log it on your chart or app. Ideally, you should track your symptoms for at least two full months. Bring your completed chart or a summary of the results to your doctor's appointment so they can review it. (Exception: If your symptoms are very bothersome, don't delay your appointment to track your symptoms.)

Question 4: Can I still have PMS or PMDD if I don't have a period every month?

Yes. It's more challenging for your doctor to make the diagnosis because she can't match your PMS/PMDD symptoms up with your period, but it is definitely possible to have PMS/PMDD without a period. This is because your ovaries (not your uterus) are in control of the large estrogen and progesterone fluctuations that cause PMS and PMDD. So regardless of what's happening with your period, if you are ovulating, PMS or PMDD is possible.

Examples of reasons you might have PMS/PMDD without having a period include: (1) you've had your uterus removed in a hysterectomy but kept your ovaries; (2) you've had an endometrial ablation, which is a procedure that helps lighten heavy periods by intentionally destroying the inside lining of the uterus (approximately 35 to 40 percent of women stop having periods after an ablation, but they still have normal ovarian function and ovulation); or (3) your periods stopped because of a progestin-containing intrauterine device (IUD) that you are using for birth control, but you're one of the 75 percent of women who still ovulate with the IUD. (Instead of consistently stopping ovulation, IUDs use other very effective techniques to prevent pregnancy).

If you don't have a monthly period, chart your symptoms to determine if they recur approximately every twenty-one to thirty-five days — if someone is ovulating every month, that's the typical number of days between periods.

Question 5: If I have it, at what age will it pop up, and when will it go away?

PMS or PMDD symptoms can start any time after you get your first period, but women in their thirties are most likely to have it, and sometimes the symptoms start to worsen as a woman gets closer to menopause. PMS resolves completely after menopause and temporarily during pregnancy or during any disruption of ovulatory cycles. (For example, your symptoms may go away if you use a type of birth control that stops you from ovulating.)

Question 6: I don't want to take hormones to treat my symptoms. But this PMS has got to go. What can I do?

If you have PMS, you can start with these fundamentals, but if you have PMDD, you should incorporate these tips while also working one-on-one with a qualified healthcare professional.

Medicine-free options for physical and emotional symptoms

- **Get exercise and relax.** Try aerobic exercise like walking, running, cycling, or swimming for at least thirty minutes a day, most days of the week (even when you don't have PMS). Also, get about eight hours of sleep each night, and participate in activities that relax you, like yoga, massage, reading, or meditation. These tips might help with fatigue, depression, and some physical symptoms.
- **Watch your diet.** To help with bloating, take it easy on the salt. And instead of eating refined sugars, eat a diet rich in complex carbohydrates. Complex carbs, such as whole-wheat pasta, sweet potatoes, brown rice, and beans enter the bloodstream gradually, causing only a moderate rise in insulin levels. This helps stabilize your mood and keep your cravings under control. Also, change your eating schedule. Eat six small meals a day rather than three large ones, or eat slightly less at

your three meals and add three light snacks throughout the day. This tip also helps symptoms by keeping
your blood-sugar level stable.

- **Try heat.** Heating pads or warm baths can help with
  cramps.
- **Limit alcohol.** A drink might seem like a good way
  to relax, but it can actually make you sleep too much,
  or it may disrupt your sleep. Both these scenarios can
  leave you feeling tired.
- **Limit caffeine.** Too much caffeine can also interfere
  with your sleep. So at the very least, avoid it four to six
  hours before bed.
- **Don't smoke.** In one large study, women who smoked
  reported more PMS symptoms and worse PMS symptoms than women who did not smoke.
- **Try acupuncture.** Some women say that acupuncture improves their mood and physical symptoms.

Traditional meds

- **Nonsteroidal anti-inflammatory drugs (NSAIDs)**
  such as ibuprofen (Motrin IB) or naproxen sodium
  (Aleve) can help reduce cramping and breast discomfort. But tell your doctor about any long-term use of
  NSAIDs because they can cause issues such as stomach ulcers.
- **Diuretics (water pills)** are drugs that lower the amount
  of salt and water in your body. Therefore, they can help
  reduce bloating and breast tenderness. If the medicine-
  free options like exercising and reducing salt intake don't
  eliminate your water retention, ask your doctor if a prescribed diuretic would be a good option for you. This
  tip is a gem that not enough people take advantage of.
  (Note: Stay well-hydrated. Limiting water intake is not
  an effective way to decrease bloating!)

Nutritional supplements and herbal remedies

Some people say that these nutritional supplements ease their PMS/PMDD symptoms, but study results are inconsistent. Here are some potential options along with a few of the symptoms they are said to help.

- **Calcium carbonate** 1,200 mg a day (may help with fatigue, cravings, and depression)
- **B_6** 50 mg a day (may help with moodiness, irritability, forgetfulness, bloating, and anxiety)
- **Magnesium** 200 to 360 mg a day (may help with bloating, mood symptoms, and migraines)
- **Polyunsaturated fatty acids** (omega-3 and omega-6) 1 to 2 g a day (may help with cramps)
- **Herbal remedies.** 20 to 40 mg of vitex agnus castus (chasteberry), a popular herbal remedy, appears to be an effective treatment option for women with mild premenstrual symptoms.[1] If you choose to use any herbal remedy, I suggest discussing the risks and benefits with your clinician. For example, St. John's Wort is commonly used, but study results regarding effectiveness are mixed, and it may reduce the effectiveness of birth control pills, and possibly the patch and ring. Also, be aware that the FDA does not regulate supplements or herbal remedies at the same level that it regulates medicines.[2]

If you try these options, don't overdo it on the dosing. For example, doses of B_6 above 100 mg a day can cause nerve damage, and high doses of calcium supplements increase your risk of kidney stones and possibly heart disease.

Of course, you could always opt for a balanced, healthy diet instead of taking a supplement.

Keep in mind that many products that are advertised to

reduce or get rid of PMS symptoms haven't been tested for safety or proven to work. So please talk with your healthcare practitioner if you have any questions.

Question 7: I'm going to need more than a nap and some vitamins. PMS/PMDD is about to have me single (or maybe even fired or in jail if my coworker doesn't back off). If my main problem is my mood, what else can I do?

An antidepressant medication called a selective serotonin reuptake inhibitor (SSRI) can be extremely helpful when it comes to mood complaints. In some cases, SSRIs help people with their physical symptoms too. Therefore, they are also an option when individuals with physical symptoms don't want to use hormonal birth control.

I typically start with fluoxetine, sertraline, citalopram, or escitalopram, since these have been studied extensively. Paroxetine is also effective, but it's more likely to cause weight gain. Once you start an SSRI, you should see some mood improvements during your first menstrual cycle, but it might take several months to get you where you want to be.

SSRIs can be taken in different regimens:

- **Continuous SSRIs.** With this option, you take an SSRI every day. This might be the best choice if your periods are irregular, you have low-level mood symptoms throughout the entire month, or you have severe physical symptoms.
- **Luteal-phase therapy.** You start taking the SSRI on the day you expect to ovulate (ovulation typically occurs approximately fourteen days before your period starts). You stop the SSRI when your period begins, or, if your symptoms continue for the first few days

of your period, you can take it during those days as well. If you have predictable symptoms that start more than a week before your period, this might be a great option for you. If you are using the SSRI to help with physical symptoms, you may need a higher dose with this regimen.

- **Symptom-onset therapy.** You start the SSRI when PMS/PMDD symptoms begin and continue until the first few days of your period. If you can easily recognize when your symptoms start, and you have symptoms for a week or less, this might be the best plan for you.

If you opt for an SSRI, you should know that some of the possible side effects include nausea, headache, decreased libido, delayed orgasm, or difficulty reaching orgasm. (If this happens to you, sexual function will return after therapy is stopped.)

To minimize the side effects, I prefer the luteal-phase or symptom-onset option (if they are effective), and I start with a low dose and slowly increase the dose as needed.

- Fluoxetine: starting dose 10 mg
- Sertraline: starting dose 12.5 mg
- Paroxetine (instant release): starting dose 10 mg
- Citalopram: starting dose 10 mg
- Escitalopram: starting dose 5 mg

If you decide to stop the SSRI after taking it continuously for several months, ask your doctor if you need to discontinue the medication gradually to avoid withdrawal symptoms.

You might have to try different SSRIs before you find the one that works best for you, but of all the treatment options for PMDD, SSRIs are the best. Up to 70 percent of symptomatic women respond to them. Marriages have literally been saved after I've prescribed these!

If anxiety is a major PMS symptom for you and the SSRIs listed above do not help, your doctor might offer you a benzodiazepine, which is an antianxiety medicine. However, this medication should be prescribed cautiously, given its potential for abuse and dependence. So if you're offered a benzodiazepine, I recommend asking for a different (nonaddictive) alternative.

Whether or not you use medication, cognitive behavioral therapy (CBT) for mood symptoms can be really helpful. And you can reach out to peer support groups.

If none of this does the trick for your mood symptoms, review the answer to question 8.

Question 8: If physical symptoms are my main complaint, or if my mood symptoms don't go away with SSRIs, what do you recommend?

Estrogen-and-progestin-containing birth control tends to help physical symptoms more than SSRIs. And some women who don't get adequate mood symptom relief with an SSRI alone will get symptom relief after switching to birth control or taking hormonal birth control in addition to their SSRI. Therefore, assuming you want birth control and it's safe for you to take estrogen, I recommend one of the following:

- Birth control pills that contain estrogen and progestin (taken daily)

   Note: Some oral birth control pills with a progestin called drospirenone are FDA approved for the treatment of physical and emotional symptoms associated with PMDD. Drospirenone may put you at a slightly higher risk for blood clots in the veins or lungs than the progestins in other pills.

- Vaginal birth control ring (a new ring is inserted at home and lasts twenty-one consecutive days)
- Birth control patch (a new patch is applied at home and lasts seven consecutive days)

When it comes to birth control for PMS or PMDD, it's important to know that although estrogen-and-progestin-containing options help a lot of women, some women find that their mood swings intensify while taking hormonal contraception. Using "monophasic birth control" (meaning each active pill delivers the same amount of estrogen and progesterone throughout the entire pill pack) decreases the chance that the birth control will worsen your mood. If you have a history of depression, make sure you tell your doctor before starting, and if your mood gets worse, tell your healthcare practitioner immediately.

If you decide to use estrogen-and-progestin-containing birth control pills, these are the regimen options:

- **Cyclic.** You have a period once a month. With this regimen, you take the estrogen-progestin (active) pills for twenty-one days, then you have a period when you take sugar pills for seven days. Alternatively, some brands of birth control pills have twenty-four days of hormones, followed by four days of sugar pills. (Note: we call them sugar pills, but sometimes they contain something beneficial, like iron.)
- **Extended cycle.** You take active pills beyond the typical twenty-one or twenty-four days. For example, if you only want to have a period every three months, you'd only take the sugar pills every three months.
- **Continuous dosing.** You don't have a period because you never take sugar pills.

You can also use the ring or patch continuously. For example, if you want to use the birth control ring continuously, remove the prior ring and insert a new one immediately every twenty-one days. To use the patch continuously, a new patch is applied every week on the same day without skipping a week. (If you decide to use the patch continuously, I recommend that you ask for the option with a lower estrogen level.)

Some patients have better symptom control when they use the extended-cycle or continuous regimens.

I usually start with estrogen-and-progestin-containing birth control, but if you don't wish to use estrogen or it's not safe for you to do so, you can also opt for a progestin-only birth control to help your physical symptoms (e.g., progestin-only intrauterine devices can help with cramps.) However, I do not recommend progestin-only birth control to treat mood symptoms.

See chapter 10 for more information about the pros and cons of different birth control options. For a list of medical conditions that make it unsafe for you to use certain birth control methods, see appendix B.

Question 9: What if none of those suggestions work?

It usually doesn't come to this, but if you have severe PMS or you have PMDD, and multiple SSRIs, birth control, and therapy don't work, or if birth control isn't an option and SSRIs and therapy don't work, your doctor might recommend a gonadotropin-releasing hormone (GnRH) agonist. By throwing your body into reversible menopause, this medication will take away the estrogen and progesterone hormonal fluctuations, which are thought to be the root cause of your symptoms. To help with menopausal symptoms like hot flashes and bone loss, your doctor can give you low-dose estrogen-progestin "add-back" therapy; however, some women may experience recurrent PMS/PMDD symptoms with the addition of these hormones.[3]

If your mood symptoms resolve with GnRH treatment, and you are able to tolerate add-back therapy, and you are finished having children, and you are several years away from natural menopause, your doctor might discuss removal of your ovaries to bring on permanent menopause. However, I want to stress that this is a last resort.

Before having the surgery, ask your doctor about the long-term risks of removing your ovaries at your age. Also, ask them to explain the pros and cons of removing your uterus at the same time.

Question 10: How long will I need to take meds to control my PMS/PMDD symptoms?

When it comes to treating PMS/PMDD, we aren't sure of the optimal length you should continue therapy. If you're using only birth control, continue it as long as you are OK with taking contraception. If you're using an SSRI, you can opt to use it indefinitely, or you can try to stop it after a year to see how you do. Or, if you are taking SSRIs continuously, another possibility is to try the luteal-phase or symptom-onset option. Then, if your symptoms return after you come off the SSRI or after you decrease how often you are taking them, you can always resume your prior treatment regimen. You can also stop your SSRI during pregnancy since PMS goes away temporarily during that time. And once you're postmenopausal, the good news is that your PMS/PMDD symptoms will resolve completely.

DR. NITA'S NOTE
Advocate for Your Health Like a Pro If You Think You Have PMS/PMDD

Here are some questions to ask your doctor:

1. *Do you think I have PMS or PMDD, or do you think something else is going on?* It is possible to have something called "premenstrual exacerbation," which is when you have an underlying condition (such as major depression, anxiety, migraines, thyroid disorder, irritable bowel syndrome, etc.) that is present all month long but gets worse during the second half of your menstrual cycle. This is why it's important to pay attention to when your symptoms are happening in relation to your period. You'll only get the right treatment if you get the right diagnosis first.

2. *Do I need labs to make sure nothing else is going on?* Your doctor might need to check your thyroid, for example.

If they confirm that you have PMS or PMDD, proceed with questions 3 through 6.

3. *Based on my history, symptoms, and contraceptive desires, which treatment option do you think I should start with, and why?* No matter what medical issue you are dealing with, it's always a good idea to ask why your doctor feels that a particular treatment or medication is the best option for you. Make sure you understand the risks of any treatment you agree to.

4. *If this doesn't work, what will we do next?* This is important because (a) if you don't improve with that

treatment option, knowing that there is a next step will help you not get discouraged. And (b) if you happen to see another doctor when you follow up, you can see if they are thinking along the same lines. If the other doctor recommends something else, that doesn't mean that either doctor is wrong. There are lots of ways to approach the treatment of PMS/PMDD. But you can ask why they prefer their treatment option instead of what the other doctor was going to do next.

5. *If my symptoms worsen, what can I do on my own? When should I contact you?* These questions are particularly important if you have mood symptoms that are associated with PMDD. If you ever have thoughts of hurting yourself or someone else, notify a healthcare practitioner immediately. Lifeline Chat is a service of the 988 Suicide & Crisis Lifeline (formerly known as the National Suicide Prevention Lifeline), connecting individuals with counselors for emotional support and other services via web chat. To speak to someone, dial 988, or go to https://988lifeline.org/chat to use the online chat option.

6. *When should I follow up with you?* Hopefully your symptoms will improve with the recommended treatment. But it's a good idea to schedule a follow up appointment just in case you need to modify your treatment plan. Make sure you continue to chart your symptoms to help determine the effectiveness of treatment.

Chapter 8

Are You Sure My Period Is Supposed to Feel Like This?

Period Pain

When it comes to period pain, many women fall into two groups. The first group is the "I've told a million doctors a million different ways that my period pain is excruciating, but nobody listens" group. These are the women who have spent way too much time curling up on the bathroom floor or crying in bed because of pain that's so intense that's all they can do. They believe either that no one can help them or that no one wants to help them. Or they've been dismissed so many times that they start to believe that they really are overreacting when it comes to their period pain ... maybe debilitating, life-sucking periods really are a natural part of womanhood, as their doctors have told them.

I call the second group period-pain warriors. These are the people who don't tell their doctor about their intense period pain because they assume it's normal. If you are in this group, please hear me when I say this: it's not! Even if your mom or your grandmother says, "Yeah, all the women in our family hurt like hell every month. That's normal for us," it's not normal. In many cases, women have or have had painful periods because of a medical condition that was never properly diagnosed and treated.

If you're in the first group, first and foremost, I apologize on behalf of every doctor who has ever dismissed you or made you feel like a liar or a drama queen. It's our job to help you, and I'm sorry if we failed you or dismissed your concerns. And if you are in the second group, please tell every reproductive-age uterus owner you know that ridiculously painful periods might be common, but that doesn't make them normal.

In this chapter I provide information that can go a long way when you are trying to figure out how to demolish your period pain.

PERIOD PAIN CRASH COURSE
What You Need to Know to Patient Like a Pro

This Q&A is for individuals who have had period pain for months or years. This info is not for those with sudden period pain or period pain that is associated with a fever.

Question 1: How do I know if my period pain is not normal? How much is too much?

Question 2: It's official, my period pain is not normal. Why do my periods hurt so bad?

Question 3: Do I have primary or secondary dysmenorrhea?

Question 4: My doctor says I don't need surgery but does think I have a gynecological reason for my pain. I don't want to take medicine. What can I do to help my primary or secondary dysmenorrhea?

Question 5: My pain laughed at those suggestions. I'm willing to be a little more aggressive, but I don't want hormones or NSAIDs. What do you recommend?

Question 6: None of that worked. What else do you have?

Question 7: I'm still hurting! Any more suggestions?

Question 8: How do I know when it's time for surgery?

Question 9: What type of surgery will I have?

Question 10: If I'm a reproductive-age woman, what should I ask if I'm told I have an ovarian cyst?

Question 1: How do I know if my period pain is not normal? How much is too much?

Normal period pain consists of mild cramping that starts a few days before your period and ends by the time your period is over. The discomfort can be controlled with self-care measures like heating pads or over-the-counter medication such as ibuprofen or naproxen sodium. Anything beyond that is too much pain. You definitely shouldn't be missing school, work, or social events because of your periods. And your period pain should not get worse as you get older.

Question 2: It's official, my period pain is not normal. Why do my periods hurt so bad?

Period pain can be separated into two categories: Primary dysmenorrhea (dis-men-or-EE-ah) and secondary dysmenorrhea, the medical terms for painful menstrual cramps.

Primary dysmenorrhea is a very common problem that is often underdiagnosed and undertreated. Here's why it happens: The lining of your uterus makes natural chemicals called *prostaglandins*. During your period, those prostaglandins make the muscles in your uterus contract (tighten up) to help shed blood and tissue. Those contractions will squeeze some of the blood vessels supplying the uterus, so you have less oxygen flowing to the uterine muscle. That's a problem because, as a general rule, the cells in your body don't enjoy being deprived of oxygen. So to let you know that it doesn't like the decreased level of oxygen flowing to your uterus, you get period pain when part of the muscle briefly loses its supply of oxygen.

Compared to people with normal, mild period cramps, people with primary dysmenorrhea have higher levels of prostaglandins in their menstrual fluid, especially during the first two days of their period. This causes uterine contractions that are abnormally strong and frequent. Translation: the pain is not "all in your head." The good news is that primary dysmenorrhea tends to lessen as you get older. It might even completely disappear if you have a baby, but we aren't certain why this happens. (Fun fact: the same prostaglandins that cause your uterus to contract also give "contract now!" messages to your intestines. Because of this, many females will notice an uptick in their pooping, or they may even have the infamous period diarrhea.)

Secondary dysmenorrhea happens … wait for it … *secondary* to an underlying physical cause. Below is a list of possible underlying conditions that can cause you to have painful periods. Some of these causes are much more common than others. More common gynecological causes of secondary dysmenorrhea are in bold. But with that said, please note that it's possible to have one of these common gynecological conditions and not have pain. For example, not all endometriosis, fibroids, or ovarian cysts cause pain.[1]

Gynecologic causes of secondary dysmenorrhea

This list is not all-inclusive, but these are a lot of the culprits.

Endometriosis: Tissue that is similar to the inside lining of the uterus (known as endometrium) is found outside the uterus.

Adenomyosis: Tissue that normally lines the uterus (endometrial tissue) grows in the muscular wall of the uterus.

Fibroids: Noncancerous growths in or on the uterus.

Ovarian cysts: Sacs filled with fluid or other tissue that form on the ovary.

Intrauterine adhesions: Scar tissue in the uterus.

Pelvic adhesions: Scar tissue outside the uterus in the pelvic region.

Chronic pelvic inflammatory disease (PID): An infection in the upper part of the genital tract, usually due to a bacterial infection that spread from the vagina or cervix into the uterus, fallopian tubes, or ovaries.

Use of an intrauterine contraceptive device (IUD): This is a type of birth control that causes dysmenorrhea in some women. (However, progestin-containing IUDs actually decrease dysmenorrhea in a lot of women.)

Pelvic congestion syndrome: Dilated pelvic veins (this is like having varicose veins around your ovaries).

Hematometra: Uterus distended with blood because of an obstruction to menstrual flow at the level of the uterus, cervix, or vagina.

Obstructive endometrial polyps: Overgrowth of cells lining the uterus (endometrium) that causes an obstruction.

Congenital obstructive Mullerian malformations: Anomalies of reproductive organ(s) that are present at birth.

Cervical stenosis: Narrowing of the lower part of the uterus.

Nongynecological problems that flare up during periods

Inflammatory bowel disease: This is a term for two conditions (Crohn's disease and ulcerative colitis) that are characterized by prolonged inflammation of the GI tract. Some symptoms include persistent diarrhea, abdominal pain, bloody stools, and weight loss.

Irritable bowel syndrome (IBS): This is a problem that affects the large intestine. It can cause abdominal cramping, bloating, and a change in bowel habits. Some people with the disorder have diarrhea. Some have constipation. Others go back and forth between the two.

Interstitial cystitis (painful bladder syndrome): This is a condition that results in an unpleasant sensation (pain, pressure, discomfort) perceived to be related to the urinary bladder.

Psychogenic disorders: Conditions such as depression, anxiety, or stress.

Unless you have an issue that happens to resolve on its own, secondary dysmenorrhea tends to worsen until you treat the underlying cause. So if you are hoping it will magically disappear if you ignore it long enough, there's a high probability that you'll be disappointed.

Question 3: Do I have primary or secondary dysmenorrhea?

Table 5 lists some questions that can point you in the right direction.

Table 5. Primary vs. Secondary Dysmenorrhea

	Primary dysmenorrhea	Secondary dysmenorrhea
When did you first notice the pain?	Usually starts in adolescence, within 1 year of your first period	Usually starts after the age of 25, but it's possible in early adolescence too[2]
When does it start and end?	Pain usually begins 1 or 2 days before you get your period or once your bleeding starts. Then the pain gradually gets better over the first 12 to 72 hours of your period.	Pain might begin a few days before your period starts. Then the pain may get worse as your period continues and might not go away after your period ends.
Does your workup (including a physical exam and imaging) show evidence of an underlying condition that could cause secondary dysmenorrhea?	No	Yes (While a physical exam and imaging are important, some causes of secondary dysmenorrhea may not be identified during a workup. Therefore, a normal physical exam and normal imaging don't definitively rule out secondary dysmenorrhea.)

If you are an adult who has period pain, I recommend that you request a transvaginal ultrasound (TVUS). During a TVUS, an ultrasound probe is inserted into your vagina to look at your uterus, ovaries, fallopian tubes, and pelvic area. Although some reasons for secondary dysmenorrhea won't be seen during a TVUS, this imaging technique will help rule out a lot of possible causes. It will also help ensure that you don't have a secondary dysmenorrhea cause that will get better only with surgery.

If you have a lot of gastrointestinal (GI) or urinary symptoms, ask your doctor if you need to see an internal medicine doctor, a family practice doctor, or a GI specialist/urologist to rule out gastrointestinal or urinary causes.

Question 4: My doctor says I don't need surgery but does think I have a gynecological reason for my pain. I don't want to take medicine. What can I do to help my primary or secondary dysmenorrhea?

Try the following:

- **Use heat.** Some studies have found that heat works as well as ibuprofen and is more effective than acet-aminophen (Tylenol). Warm baths, heating pads, or hot water bottles can all help.
- **Exercise.** Exercising most days of the week can make you feel better. Aerobic workouts, such as walking, jogging, biking, or swimming, help stimulate the release of endorphins (the body's natural painkillers).
- **Try relaxation techniques.** Yoga or an abdominal or lower-back massage might decrease your pain.

Even if these suggestions don't resolve your period pain, they can improve the effectiveness of other treatments.

Question 5: My pain laughed at those suggestions. I'm willing to be a little more aggressive, but I don't want hormones or NSAIDs. What do you recommend?

- **High-frequency transcutaneous electrical nerve stimulation (TENS).** This inexpensive, noninvasive, medicine-free option works wonders for a lot of patients, especially when used in conjunction with the hormones and NSAIDs that are recommended in question 6. TENS involves attaching electrodes to the painful areas on your abdomen or lower back. The electrodes deliver small electrical currents to the body, which you'll feel as a tingling, vibrating, or muscle-twitching sensation. TENS devices can be worn discreetly under clothes as you go about your daily activities. We believe that the device works by altering the body's ability to receive and perceive pain signals rather than having a direct effect on uterine contractions. This treatment has minimal risks and few contraindications, so it's definitely worth a try.

  Some TENS devices require a prescription, but others can be purchased online or at pharmacies without a prescription. If you purchase one, it's important to have the correct settings: The pulse frequency should be between 50 and 120 Hz, since this is the range that is effective for period pain. Also, gradually increase the device's intensity level until an intense *but comfortable* sensation is achieved.

- **Pelvic floor physical therapy.** The pain caused by dysmenorrhea can make you clench your pelvic muscles so much that they end up being chronically tight and tender. So if your insurance will pay for it, I'm a *huge* fan of pelvic floor physical therapy (PT), especially when used in conjunction with the hormones and NSAIDs that are recommended in question 6. A pelvic physical therapist can teach you how to relax your pelvic muscles (and any other surrounding muscles or tissues that may also be causing or contributing to your pain), and that can help your discomfort a lot. These PT sessions last about an hour and are usually once to twice weekly. But it typically takes months to feel better, so don't give up too soon. Also, know that you may temporarily experience an increased amount of pain when you first start PT as your muscles become "reeducated."

If pelvic physical therapy doesn't get you the relief you need or if you can't tolerate PT because you have too much discomfort, you might benefit from trigger-point injections. This is when medication designed to relieve pain is injected directly into your problematic muscles. The procedure takes about twenty to thirty minutes, and the pain relief may last anywhere from a few hours up to a few months. Then, repeat injections may be needed. Or occasionally a woman's pain may completely resolve without additional injections.

You can also try these suggestions, but we don't have enough research for me to confidently say they will effectively treat your period pain:

- **Vitamin B1** 100 mg daily
- **Vitamin B6** 100 mg daily (doses above 100 mg a day can cause nerve damage)
- **Magnesium** (optimal dose or regimen not known)
- **Daily fish oil supplements** with 1,080 mg eicosapentaenoic acid and 720 mg docosahexaenoic acid daily
- **Ginger powder** 750 to 2,000 mg on days one to three of your period

- **Low-fat vegetarian diet**
- **Acupuncture or acupressure**

Some people recommend Vitamin E or Vitamin D. However, I excluded them from this list due to potential safety concerns with the doses recommended to treat dysmenorrhea.

DR. NITA'S NOTE
Endometriosis Spotlight

What is endometriosis (endo)? It's when tissue that is similar to the inside lining of the uterus is found outside the uterus — where it should not be. When this tissue grows, it causes inflammation, which can lead to pain and adhesions.

Why does it happen? There are multiple proposed theories, but we don't know the exact cause of endometriosis.

How common is it? It's the most common cause of secondary dysmenorrhea. About 1 out of every 10 women of reproductive age has endometriosis, and up to 50 percent of women with infertility have it. Having an affected first-degree relative increases your risk by seven to ten times, but having a more distant relative with endo, such as a cousin, also increases your risk. And remember that it can be inherited from your mother's or your father's side.

Endo is especially common among women in their thirties or forties, but it can occur in adolescents who have just started to have their periods.

What are the symptoms? Many people don't have any symptoms at all. Others can't get out of bed when their endo flares up. When symptoms are present, they can be all over the place. The most common include pain with periods, abdominal or pelvic pain between periods, painful sex, or heavy periods. Additionally, if endometriosis affects the bowel or bladder, there can be pain with defecating or urinating, respectively (especially during periods). Occasionally, endo can also occur outside the pelvis. Some women with lung/diaphragm endometriosis, for example, might complain of chest or shoulder pain. And to make things even more confusing, the timing of any of these symptoms can vary. Some women constantly have them, but others only experience them with periods or around the time of ovulation.

Since symptoms can vary so much, it takes a woman an average of eight to twelve years to get a diagnosis after their symptoms start.

How is it diagnosed? We can strongly suspect endometriosis based on symptoms and the results of imaging we order, but there isn't a blood test, urine test, or imaging study that can help doctors make the definitive diagnosis. The only way to know for sure that you have endo is by having a surgery to see and test (biopsy) the abnormal tissue. The surgery is usually done laparoscopically, which means a small cut is made (usually near your belly button) and a slender camera is inserted to look at your pelvis and abdomen. During surgery, your doctor will determine if your endometriosis is stage 1 (minimal endometriosis), stage 2, stage 3, or stage 4 (a lot of endometriosis). However, the amount of endo seen during surgery doesn't always correspond to the amount of pain a person is having. For instance, you may have a lot of pain with stage 1 endometriosis or minimal pain with stage 4 endo.

How can my endometriosis be treated? Treatment for endometriosis typically involves medication and/or surgery. To avoid potential complications (such as adhesions that can form even if surgery is performed perfectly), I recommend that you opt for medication instead of surgery when possible.

Medications

The medicine listed in this section will not improve fertility or treat endometriosis that is causing a blockage in one of your organs (e.g., your bowel). Additionally, meds are also un-likely to resolve an endometrioma, which is an ovarian cyst containing endometriosis tissue. Surgery is the appropriate way to treat these issues. (Exception: small endometriomas that are not causing a lot of pain may be monitored.)

In addition to suppressing your symptoms, hormonal medication may help slow the growth of endometriosis and keep new adhesions from forming. But these drugs aren't designed to get rid of endometriosis tissue that is already there. In other words, medication doesn't cure endometrio-sis. If your pain does decrease on meds, once you stop them, your symptoms are very likely to return.

Here's a quick rundown of some medication options.

- Hormonal birth control containing estrogen and pro-gestin. I recommend a continuous birth control regimen (meaning you take active hormones continuously to prevent your period from coming). Compared to cyclic or extended regimens, this may do a better job at pre-venting the growth of new endo. Doing what you can to prevent the progression of endo is important for pain relief and also for future fertility. See chapter 10 for more info on birth control regimens.
- Progestin-only hormonal birth control. These hor-monal options include progestin-containing intrauter-ine devices (IUDs), the birth control shot, the birth control implant, or progestin-only birth control pills.
- Norethindrone acetate. This is a progestin-only pill, but this medication is not labeled for contraception. A com-monly used regimen of norethindrone acetate is 5 mg by mouth daily, but your practitioner may increase the

dose to 15 mg daily depending on side effects including breakthrough bleeding.

- Nonsteroidal anti-inflammatory drugs (NSAIDs). This includes nonprescription, over-the-counter pain relievers such as ibuprofen or naproxen. If over-the-counter NSAIDs don't provide relief, your doctor may prescribe a higher dose. Starting these medications one to two days before your period works best to reduce menstrual pain. NSAIDs are frequently used in addition to hormonal medications, such as birth control.

- Gonadotropin-releasing hormone (GnRH) antagonist or GnRH agonist. This is an option if birth control, norethindrone acetate, and NSAIDs don't provide relief. These meds work by temporarily suppressing ovarian estrogen production. This causes the endometriosis tissue to shrink, reducing pain in more than 80 percent of people, including those with severe pain. However, the downside is that your decreased estrogen levels may lead to significant side effects such as decreased bone mineral density (weakening of the bones), hot flashes, and vaginal dryness. One way to minimize these side effects is to take hormonal "add-back" treatment (adding very small amounts of estrogen or progestin) in addition to the GnRH medication. But due to concerns about weakening of the bones over time, current recommendations are that GnRH agonists only be used for up to 12 months. With once-daily dosing, antagonists can be used for up to 24 months. (I recommend a GnRH antagonist instead of an agonist; unlike GnRH agonists, these agents are effective immediately. GnRH antagonists are available in both oral and injectable forms.) Of note, these meds are very expensive if you don't have insurance coverage.

- In severe, difficult-to-treat cases, your doctor might

recommend an aromatase inhibitor. These drugs block a specific enzyme (aromatase) that increases estrogen levels in tissue. This may be helpful because there's increasing evidence that endometriosis tissue makes its own aromatase. However, we need more research before this option is routinely recommended.

Surgery

Don't be in a rush to have surgery if it's not necessary. It's best to try to control your symptoms with lifestyle modifications and medications first. Reasons to have surgery include infertility, a large endometrioma, extreme pain, moderate pain that isn't responding to medication, or because the endometriosis is causing a blockage in one of your organs (e.g., your bowel).

The goal of surgery is to remove endometriosis and scar tissue. When considering surgery for pelvic endo, here are some tips:

- Sometimes your options are limited when it comes to picking a surgeon because of insurance. But if you can, I strongly recommend finding someone who does a lot of endometriosis surgery. Why? Some endo can be hard to detect, and some of the lesions can be tricky to remove. You want someone who is really good at doing this surgery.
- When you have surgery for endometriosis, the goal is to destroy all the endo that is seen. Before your surgery, make sure you ask your surgeon this question: "If you see endometriosis, will you burn it or cut it out?" Some doctors will do what's called an ablation. That basically uses heat to burn off the top layer of

the endometriosis lesion, but the burn might not go deep enough to get rid of it all. Ideally, you want a doctor who will resect (cut out) the endometriosis if it's in a location that's safe to cut. In other words, ablation removes surface, easily visible endo. Excision cuts as deep as needed to remove all your endometriosis. Both ablation and excision are performed laparoscopically, meaning a tiny camera is inserted in the navel, but some surgeons are more skilled at excision (which is a more difficult surgery to perform). You want a surgeon who is skilled at excision procedures.

- If you are having an endometrioma removed, ask if they will excise the entire endometrioma or just stick a needle in it to drain it. Excision is superior to drainage. (But note that surgery on the ovary will diminish its ability to produce eggs over time.)

- Ask your doctor if they are concerned about bladder endo. If so ask if they think you'd benefit from a cystoscopy, which is when a lighted camera is inserted into your bladder to inspect the bladder walls.

- Approximately 75 percent of people who have this surgery have less pain for several months after the procedure. However, up to 8 in 10 women have pain again within two years of surgery. Having an experienced surgeon who resects your endometriosis instead of ablating it and using meds such as a progestin IUD after surgery will increase the chance that you'll stay pain-free for longer. (Tip: If your doctor recommends an IUD, you can ask them to put it in while you are asleep in the operating room. That will save you the discomfort of an office IUD insertion.)

- If you don't desire a future pregnancy, your doctor might recommend a hysterectomy (removal of the uterus) with or without an oophorectomy (removal of the ovaries).

If both of your ovaries are removed, your body will no longer produce estrogen and you will officially be menopausal. Symptoms may recur in women even after hysterectomy and oophorectomy. This may be because of endometriosis that was missed during surgery.

- If you are interested in learning more about this condition, I recommend the book *Beating Endo* by Dr. Iris Kerin Orbuch and Amy Stein.

Additional Suggestions That May Help

- TENS and/or pelvic physical therapy with or without trigger point injections may help with pain (see question 5 for more details).
- Watch your diet. There isn't a specific diet that will prevent or cure endometriosis. However, endometriosis is an inflammatory process. So it makes sense that you shouldn't eat foods that promote inflammation. Some common inflammatory foods include French fries and other fried foods, soda and other sugar-sweetened beverages, red meat (burgers, steaks), processed meat (sausage, hot dogs), and refined carbohydrates such as white bread and pastries. I'm not saying that you have to give up everything forever. This will be a trial-and-error process. Give up inflammatory foods for a few weeks, then add those foods back into your diet one at a time. If your symptoms flare up, you'll know that a particular food group might be problematic for you. Anti-inflammatory foods like olive oil, tomatoes, green leafy vegetables (such as spinach, kale, and collards), fruits (such as strawberries, blueberries, cherries, and oranges), and fatty fish (like salmon, mackerel, tuna, and sardines) all work to counteract inflammation.

- Beware of endocrine disruptors. Endocrine disruptors are hormone imitators that trick your body into thinking they're natural hormones. These chemicals are linked with developmental, reproductive, brain, immune, and other problems, such as cancer. Endocrine disruptors, such as phthalates and bisphenol A (BPA) can be found in everything from plastic bottles, food containers, and liners of metal food cans to toys, cosmetics, and even food. I recommend that you google endocrine disruptors to learn more about where they are found. We are still learning about how exposure to endocrine disruptors might be linked to endometriosis.
- Auricular (ear) acupuncture. Acupuncture needles are inserted at specific points on the outer ear. According to some research this helps relieve pain. It's worth a shot!
- See a therapist if needed. I'm not recommending this because you are imagining the pain, but because dealing with a chronic issue like endometriosis can take an emotional toll and lead to depression and anxiety. Therapy won't cure your endometriosis, but it can help with the emotional difficulties that come with it.

Question 6: None of that worked. What else do you have?

There's not a set rule when it comes to the order, but ask your practitioner about mixing and matching these three options:

- **Hormones.** This includes estrogen-and-progestin-containing birth control pills, the vaginal ring, or the transdermal patch. You can also opt for a progestin-only birth control option, including progestin-only birth control pills, the birth control shot, the implant, or a progestin-containing IUD. I've seen great results with progestin-containing IUDs, and the birth control shot also works well for a lot of people with dysmenorrhea. But birth control isn't one-size-fits-all, so you might have to try a few options before you figure out what works best for you. If you choose the pill, vaginal ring, or patch, I recommend extended-cycle or continuous birth control, meaning you only have a period every few months or you never have a period. (No period equals no pain for a lot of women.) See chapter 10 for more info on birth control options.

Another hormonal option that you can use is norethindrone acetate. You can start at 5 mg once daily, and your doctor can slowly increase the dose to reach 15 mg a day, if needed. This medication is an oral progestin, but it is not labeled as birth control.

- **NSAIDs (like ibuprofen or naproxen sodium).** Whether you have primary or secondary dysmenorrhea, it helps to get ahead of the pain with NSAIDs. Sometimes, if a patient is having a tough time controlling their period pain with over-the-counter strength NSAIDs, I increase the dosage. For prescription level dosing, I recommend taking ibuprofen 600 to 800 mg by mouth every eight hours, starting twenty-four hours before your period is scheduled to start. I then instruct patients to continue taking the med every eight hours for the first forty-eight to seventy-two hours of their period. (Or, for unpredictable periods, the medication is initiated on the first day of bleeding and continued on a scheduled basis for two or three days.)

If you don't respond to ibuprofen, you may have better luck with another oral NSAID called mefenamic acid. I recommend 500 mg by mouth when symptoms start, then 250 mg every six hours for two or three days.

But make sure you check in with your doctor before taking prescription-level doses. And to decrease the chance of gastrointestinal side effects, take your NSAIDs with food.

Women with asthma, bleeding disorders, aspirin allergy, liver damage, stomach disorders, or ulcers should not take NSAIDs.

- **Acetaminophen (Tylenol).** If a patient can't tolerate NSAIDs for any reason, Tylenol can be used instead, but it doesn't tend to work as well as NSAIDs for period pain.

Again, there isn't a set way to mix and match these three options. For instance, you can try birth control first or NSAIDs first, or you can use them simultaneously from the start. Regardless of what you choose, if you don't see improvement in your pain after three or four months, it's time to switch things up (even if switching things up simply means trying a different birth control or NSAID option).

Question 7: I'm still hurting! Any more suggestions?

If you haven't given pelvic physical therapy or TENS a try, I'd urge you to reconsider (see question 5).

GnRH antagonist or agonist. If the suggestions listed in question 6 don't help, this is another option. GnRH antagonists and GnRH agonists are two medications that basically throw your body into fake, reversible menopause. These options cause menopause-like side effects such as hot flashes, and they are very expensive if you don't have insurance coverage. They also cause loss of bone density (bone weakness) with prolonged use. Your doctor can give you small amounts of estrogen and progesterone to offset the bone loss and menopause-related symptoms, but due to the impact on bones, most clinicians only prescribe this treatment for a limited time. (Current recommendations limit the use of GnRH agonists for up to twelve months. Depending on the dosing, some GnRH antagonists can be taken for up to twenty-four months.) Taking continuous combined hormonal contraception or using a progestin-only birth control (like an IUD or Depo-Provera) after stopping the GnRH medication may result in a prolonged pain-free period.

If you are close to menopause or if you need to put off surgery for a while, a GnRH agonist or antagonist may be a great choice for you.

Question 8: How do I know when it's time for surgery?

If your doctor sees a reason for secondary dysmenorrhea on imaging that they know won't get better with the nonsurgical options listed above, then they'll recommend surgery without trying medication first. But in situations when surgery is not needed immediately, I *strongly* recommend that you give NSAIDs and/or hormonal treatment a try for six months. Then, if you're not feeling better, surgery might be the best next step to either (a) see if there is a cause for secondary dysmenorrhea that wasn't seen on imaging or (b) treat the known cause for secondary dysmenorrhea that didn't get better with medication. But a six-month time frame isn't a hard-and-fast rule. Depending on how much your pain disrupts your life, you might choose to have surgery sooner, you might put it off for longer than six months while you try a variety of nonsurgical treatment options, or you might choose never to have surgery.

Your doctor might also have reasons for suggesting that you wait longer than six months (for example, if you are at a high risk for surgical complications). However, if your doctor wants you to wait longer but you feel like the intensity of your pain makes surgery the most appropriate next step, you should definitely get a second opinion.

Question 9: What type of surgery will I have?

That depends on the cause of your pain and whether you want to have kids in the future. Some common surgical options include the following:

For people who want (or possibly want) to have children

- Your doctor might recommend a surgery called a diagnostic laparoscopy. That's when they make one or two small incisions in your abdomen and insert a camera to look for any abnormalities that could be causing your pain. If they see an underlying reason for secondary dysmenorrhea during the operation (like endometriosis), they can address it during the surgery. Some causes of pain can be corrected through vaginal procedures (without the need for laparoscopy).

For people who are absolutely, positively sure they don't want to carry a pregnancy in the future

- **Hysterectomy.** This is surgical removal of the uterus (depending on your age and the cause of your dysmenorrhea, removal of your ovaries might also be recommended).
- **Endometrial ablation.** This procedure, which is done through the vagina, removes or destroys the inside lining of the uterus. It is usually done to help with heavy periods, but in one study, about half of people who had dysmenorrhea that was related to heavy

menstrual bleeding said that their period pain resolved after an ablation was performed. However, before having an ablation to decrease pain, you should ask your doctor how confident they are that the procedure will be helpful. An endometrial ablation will *not* resolve pain for many causes of secondary dysmenorrhea.

As long as both of your ovaries are not removed during the surgeries, the procedures above will not cause you to become menopausal.

Question 10: If I'm a reproductive-age woman, what should I ask if I'm told I have an ovarian cyst?

Does the cyst look cancerous?

When a reproductive age woman is told they have an ovarian cyst, a lot of them will worry about it being cancer. The probability of cancer does increase with age (e.g., a fifty-year-old is more likely to have ovarian cancer than a twenty-year-old), but in most cases, the answer to this question will be no. (See the ovarian cancer section on pages 261–62 for more info.)

What type of cyst is it?

Types of cysts include the following:

- **Functional cyst.** During the beginning of a normal menstrual cycle, a small cyst forms to house your maturing egg. Then, around the middle of your menstrual cycle, you ovulate, which means the egg pops out of the ovary and goes into the fallopian tube to meet up with the sperm. After the egg is released, the cyst wall usually goes away. But if all those steps don't go as planned, you can get one of these two types of functional cysts:

- **Follicular cyst.** This type occurs when a sac on the ovary doesn't release an egg and the sac swells up with fluid.
- **Corpus luteum cyst.** This type occurs when the sac releases an egg, then reseals and fills with fluid.

  Functional cysts, which are the most common type of ovarian cysts, usually don't cause symptoms, and they often go away without treatment within six to eight weeks.

- **Teratoma (dermoid).** This cyst contains different kinds of tissues that make up the body, such as skin, hair, or teeth. Teratomas may be present from birth and can grow during the reproductive years. In very rare cases, some teratomas can become cancerous.
- **Cystadenoma.** This is a cyst that forms on the outer surface of the ovary. These tumors can grow very large, but they usually are benign.
- **Endometrioma.** This cyst forms as a result of endometriosis. Endometriomas are usually filled with old blood that resembles chocolate syrup; therefore, they are sometimes called "chocolate cysts."

Women with polycystic ovarian syndrome (PCOS), which is a common condition caused by an imbalance of reproductive hormones, may have many small cysts. These cysts do not cause pain or need to be removed, but these women may need treatment for other PCOS problems, such as irregular menstrual periods. For more on PCOS, see the spotlight on page 208.

Do you think this cyst is causing my pain?

Most cysts don't cause symptoms. For example, an unruptured two-centimeter follicular cyst is not a likely cause of pain. However, some cysts may cause a dull or sharp ache in the abdomen and pain during certain activities. Also, cysts that bleed or burst also may cause sudden, severe pain. And large cysts may cause your ovary to twist. This twisting, which is called an ovarian torsion, may cause pain on one side that comes and goes or can start suddenly.

Most ovarian cysts go away within a few months without any treatment. But if a cyst is large or causing symptoms or if cancer is suspected, surgery may be recommended. If you have an ovarian torsion, you need surgery immediately.

Do I need repeat imaging to make sure the cyst resolves? If so, when?

Many cysts do not require repeat imaging, but sometimes repeat imaging is recommended after two to three months to reevaluate the cyst.

If you repeatedly get cysts, hormonal birth control may be recommended. The birth control won't make your current cyst resolve faster, but it *might* prevent new cysts from forming. See chapter 10 for more information regarding the use of hormonal contraception for ovarian cyst prevention.

DR. NITA'S NOTE
Advocate for Your Health Like a Pro When You Have Period Pain

Here are some questions to ask your doctor:

• *Do you think I have primary dysmenorrhea or secondary dysmenorrhea?* Tip: The word *dysmenorrhea* is a mouthful. If you feel uncomfortable saying the word, you can simply ask if they think your pain is due to an underlying cause. Or you can google the word and use the speaking feature on your phone or computer to hear how to pronounce it.

If they think you have primary dysmenorrhea, ask:

- *What treatment do you recommend?* Make sure you understand the treatment plan, and ask when you should follow up.

    If your pain resolves, great! You're all set.

    If your pain doesn't resolve, here are a couple of tips:

    If your doctor didn't initially order imaging, I recommend that you request a transvaginal ultrasound to help ensure that secondary dysmenorrhea isn't to blame. (Remember, primary dysmenorrhea usually starts within a year of your first period.)

    As far as adjusting your treatment plan, it really depends on how bothersome your dysmenorrhea is and what you desire. You can try different pill-free options as long as you'd like. But once you add NSAIDs/hormones into the mix, I recommend that you check in with your doctor if your pain persists in spite of three to four months of taking the meds as prescribed. At that time, they may make a small adjustment or totally change your treatment plan. If your pain persists in spite of NSAIDs/hormonal birth control, which are known to help primary dysmenorrhea, it's likely that you have secondary dysmenorrhea.

If they think you have secondary dysmenorrhea, ask:

1. *Will you order imaging to confirm the diagnosis?* If a patient's only period complaint is dysmenorrhea, ob-gyns frequently order a transvaginal ultrasound. However, if your doctor is concerned about other problems, they may suggest other imaging, such as a CT scan, an MRI, or a more specialized type of ultrasound that involves putting a small amount of saline in your uterus.

Imaging doesn't definitively rule out every possible cause of period pain, but it helps us put the pieces of the puzzle together.

2. *I have a family history of (insert the secondary cause(s) of dysmenorrhea that run(s) in your family). Does that increase my risk of having that (those) condition(s)?* Having a family history of something doesn't automatically mean you will have that condition, but depending on what it is, it might increase your odds. Therefore, if nothing else, this question motivates your practitioner to take your family history into account.

3. *Do you think I need to see another type of doctor to rule out nongynecologic reasons for the pain?* Remember that you can have more than one issue going on. If you have frequent constipation and diarrhea in addition to your period pain, for example, they might want you to see a GI doctor. Having your ob-gyn and GI doctor work you up at the same time will help you get the answers you need faster. If they want you to see another doctor, ask if they recommend a specific person.

4. *What treatment should I proceed with while we are doing the workup?* Make sure you understand the plan.

5. *When should I follow up with you to review the imaging result?* At your follow-up appointment, they may be able to give you a definitive diagnosis. But just in case they can't, go to your appointment with this backup plan: Copy the list of possible causes of secondary dysmenorrhea in question 2 (page 157), and bring it to your follow-up appointment. If they are unsure of your diagnosis, say something like, "I know we are still trying to determine the cause of my pain, but I'd love to know what has been ruled out. Could you

look at this list and put a star by the ones you think could be the cause? Or, if you think my pain is due to something not on the list, can you write it at the bottom?" Then, each time you return, bring your list back to see if more potential causes can be excluded as your workup progresses. This will allow you to do a more focused Google search on reputable websites to help you understand your treatment options. There is a list of reputable resources at the end of the book.

6. *What treatment should I proceed with now, and when should I follow up again?* If you try a particular medication regimen, you should see improvement in three to four months. If not, ask if your treatment plan can be reevaluated. See question 8 (page 173) for a discussion of when surgery might be appropriate.

A few extra #DrNitaNotes

•   Imaging is great, but it has its limitations. There is a chance that your symptoms will improve or resolve before you get a definitive diagnosis. For instance, say that based on your symptoms, your doctor thinks you have endometriosis. If she can control your endometriosis symptoms with hormonal birth control, she might say, "Based on everything I know, I think you might have endometriosis. But since I can control your pain and you are not currently dealing with infertility, I don't recommend taking you to surgery to get a definitive diagnosis at this time."

•   Whether you're dealing with primary or secondary dysmenorrhea, if you end up following up several times to try different medication options, always ask your doctor to review your medication list to determine whether you can stop taking any of the meds that haven't worked.

- If you are one of the 50 to 90 percent of women who report painful menstrual periods, I'll be honest: It might take some time to determine what's causing your pain, and you might have to try different treatment options before you figure out the best one for you. And, unfortunately, not every doctor will have the patience to take that journey with you.

  But this is for sure: your doctor should rule out other possible causes before saying your pain is due to psychogenic (mental or emotional) reasons.

- Your dysmenorrhea is not adequately treated until your period pain no longer disrupts your daily life.

Chapter 9

Period Chaos

Periods That Are Heavy, Irregular, or Missing in Action

Me: "How are your periods?"

New patient: "They're fine."

Me (being skeptical because I know that women tend to downplay their periods, even when their underwear looks like a slaughterhouse floor every month): "Describe a typical period."

New patient: "The first three days I always wear a tampon and an extra-large pad. At night, I still double up on protection, and I set my alarm for 3 a.m. to change, but I still end up with blood-stained sheets sometimes." The patient continues to nonchalantly give a two-minute monologue that includes scenarios like sitting on the edge of chairs and holding in sneezes during her period because she lives in a constant state of fear that she'll bleed through her clothes.

Me: Do you have an urge to eat nonfood items like ice, dirt, paper, paint chips, or baby powder?

New patient (with a friendly side-eye): "How did you know that?"

Me: Pica is an eating disorder that involves craving nonfood items like the ones I mentioned. People with heavy periods frequently have pica due to iron-deficiency anemia.

Although I had to coax the information out of her, I want to point out the fact that her description of her situation was superb. If you have heavy or irregular periods, don't just say, "I have heavy periods." A busy doctor might easily dismiss that statement. Instead, tell a descriptive story about the things you avoid or the ways that your period has caused stress or embarrassment. If you bled through your clothes at a work meeting recently, say that. If your period is so heavy that you sit on a blanket when you're driving, say that. If you always have to wear some type of period protection "just in case" your irregular period decides to randomly pop up, or if you are tired of saying RIP to underwear, tell your practitioner. Tell your story! We won't know that you are being tormented by your period unless you tell us.

In regard to this new patient, we were able to quickly identify and treat the cause of her bleeding, and she moved on with her life. And I'm confident that a lot of you reading this book can have a similar success story!

Whether your periods are extremely heavy and frequent or they disappear for months at a time, these are my top ten questions and answers to prep you for your appointment.

PERIOD CHAOS CRASH COURSE
What You Need to Know to Patient Like a Pro

This information is for nonpregnant, reproductive aged adults — meaning adults who are at an age when they can get pregnant naturally. Additionally, we are only focusing on the treatment options for nonemergent causes of heavy, irregular periods.

Question 1: How do I know if I have a heavy or irregular period that I need to tell my doctor about?

Question 2: I have too much bleeding. Why are my periods out of whack?

Question 3: How can I find out if I have fibroids, adenomyosis, or polyps?

Question 4: How can I find out if I have endometrial cancer or precancer?

Question 5: My doctor confirmed that I have one of those growths. What are some treatment options I should ask about?

Question 6: We checked, and my doctor said I don't have a growth. Why else might my periods be heavy or irregular?

Question 7: Aside from a growth and ovulation problems, what's another possible cause of heavy/irregular bleeding that I should look out for?

Question 8: What are some other possible causes for heavy, irregular periods?

Question 9: Could my bleeding be due to more than one cause?

Question 10: We've talked a lot about adults who bleed too much, but aside from PCOS, what are some other reasons an adult might have a period that's missing in action?

Question 1: How do I know if I have a heavy or irregular period that I need to tell my doctor about?

If you fall into either of the following categories, you should tell your healthcare practitioner so they can evaluate you for *abnormal uterine bleeding* (AUB), which is a fancy way to say that something about your menstrual cycle is out of whack.

Category 1: You have too much bleeding.

- Periods that are super heavy
  - Bleeding that soaks through one or more tampons or pads every hour for several hours in a row
  - Menstrual flow with blood clots that are as big as a quarter or larger
  - Needing to double up on protection to control menstrual flow
  - Having to change pads or tampons during the night
  - Bleeding that is heavy enough to disrupt your daily life (for example, you miss work or a party because of your heavy flow)
- Periods that last too long: Bleeding that lasts longer than seven days
- Bleeding that comes too often
  - Having two periods less than twenty-one days apart (You should have at least twenty-one days between periods. In other words, if you have a period on the first of the month, you can have another one that starts twenty-one days later — that same month — and still fall within the normal range.)
- Spotting that pops up between your regular periods
- Periods that are heavy or frequent enough to cause iron-deficiency anemia: Blood contains iron. So if you lose a lot of blood, you lose a lot of iron, and that can cause iron-deficiency anemia, which is when your lack of iron leads to you not having enough healthy red blood cells to carry adequate oxygen to your body's organs. People with anemia may notice symptoms such as fatigue, weakness, pale skin, shortness of breath, dizziness, thinning hair, cold hands and feet, chest pain, or an irregular heartbeat.

Pica, which was mentioned in the chapter intro,

can be linked to a lot of medical issues. However, pagophagia (pag-uh-FAY-jee-uh), pica specifically focused on chewing ice, is considered to be very specific to iron deficiency. If a person increases their iron level with oral iron or iron infusions, they usually stop craving ice.

Category 2: The length of time between your periods keeps changing.

Your menstrual cycle is counted from the first day of one menstrual period to the first day of your next period. Normal menstrual cycles are between twenty-one and thirty-five days. If the number of days between an adult's periods varies by more than seven to nine days, their periods are irregular.

DR. NITA'S NOTE
Heavy or Irregular Period Cheat Sheet

There is a lot of information in this chapter. So to help guide you, I created this cheat sheet to summarize the common culprits. If you have heavy or irregular periods, these are some causes I want you to consider. Each of these possibilities will be discussed in detail in this chapter.

- **Fibroids.** Benign growths in or on the uterus
- **Adenomyosis.** The inside lining of the uterus (endometrium) grows into the wall of the uterus
- **Polyps.** Ball-like overgrowths of the endometrium
- **Endometrial cancer/precancer.** Cancer or precancer of the inside lining of the uterus (endometrium)
- **Anovulation.** Ovulation is when you release an egg from your ovary during your menstrual cycle; anovulation is when this doesn't happen.

- **Bleeding disorder.** When a woman's blood doesn't clot properly, it can lead to heavy, irregular bleeding.
- **Other.** This is where I list other issues you should know about that don't fit into one of the categories above. Topics covered include perimenopause, cesarean scar defects, medications you are taking, a problem with your endometrial lining, or just being lucky (I guess).

Question 2: I have too much bleeding. Why are my periods out of whack?

One possible reason for your abnormal uterine bleeding is that you are one of the millions of uterus owners who has something growing in their uterus that shouldn't be there. Here are some possible culprits.

- **Fibroids** (also known as leiomyomas, pronounced lie-oh-my-OH-mas, or myomas). These are growths in or on the muscular wall of the uterus. Periods may be heavy and long, and you may have vaginal spotting between periods. The bleeding may get worse over time.

  This is important: fibroids can be *submucosal* (protruding into the uterine cavity, growing where a baby typically grows during pregnancy), *intramural* (in the uterine wall), or *subserosal* (on the outer surface of the uterus); see figure 7. Fibroids that are totally or mostly submucosal frequently cause heavy and/or irregular periods. Large intramural fibroids may lead to heavy/irregular periods as well as pelvic pain. Subserosal fibroids typically don't cause heavy or irregular bleeding, but they can cause severe pelvic pain if they put pressure on the surrounding organs. Some fibroids are so big that they extend from the serosa to the submucosa.

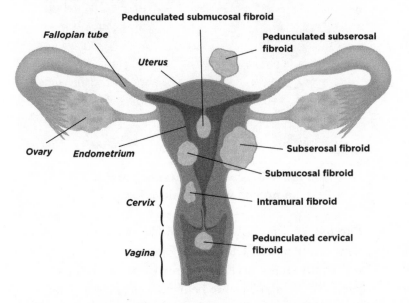

Figure 7. Types of uterine fibroids

When a submucosal or subserosal fibroid is on a thin stalk, it is called a "pedunculated fibroid." If the stalk happens to become twisted, these fibroids can become painful.

A woman may only have one fibroid, or she may have any combination of these types. Fibroids may be smaller than a pea or as large as a watermelon.

Rarely (less than one in one thousand) a cancerous fibroid will occur. This is called a leiomyosarcoma (LIE-oh-MY-oh-sar-co-ma).

- **Adenomyosis** (ad-no-my-OH-sis). With this noncancerous condition, the cells in the lining of the uterus (endometrium) grow into the muscular wall of the uterus; see figure 8. People frequently complain of heavy, painful periods that continue to get worse over time.

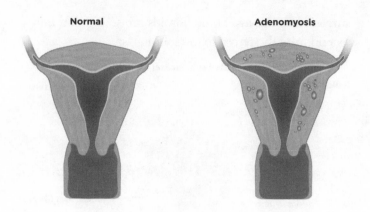

**Figure 8. A normal uterus versus
a uterus with adenomyosis**

- **Polyps.** Uterine polyps are ball-like overgrowths of
  the endometrium. They can be attached to the inner
  wall of the uterus, or they can arise from the cervix (see
  figure 9). Most polyps are benign (noncancerous), but
  some can be cancerous or precancerous (meaning they
  could eventually turn into cancer, if not treated).

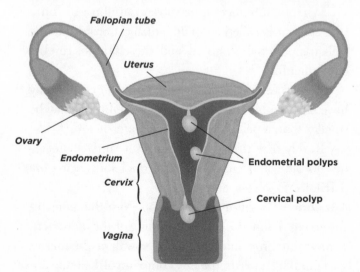

Figure 9. Endometrial and cervical polyps

- **Endometrial cancer or precancer.** This is cancer or precancer of the inside lining of the uterus (endometrium). Obesity and irregular periods are two common risk factors for these conditions. (Instead of saying, "precancer," your doctor may use the terms *endometrial hyperplasia with atypia* or *endometrial intraepithelial neoplasia*.)

Question 3: How can I find out if I have fibroids, adenomyosis, or polyps?

To check for fibroids, adenomyosis, or polyps, your practitioner may offer you a transvaginal ultrasound (TVUS). During that procedure, an ultrasound probe is inserted into your vagina to look at your uterus, ovaries, and fallopian tubes. While transvaginal ultrasounds are frequently recommended, they miss one out of six growths in the uterus in reproductive-aged women. That means that one out of six women will be told, "Everything looks great!" when everything is *not* great. Therefore, if cost and availability are not an issue for you, I recommend that you ask if you're a good candidate for saline infusion sonography (SIS) instead. This procedure, which is frequently performed in gynecology clinics, is just like a regular transvaginal ultrasound, except that saline is used to gently expand the walls of your uterus and hold them apart. Compared to a transvaginal ultrasound, the SIS allows your doctor to get a better view of the uterine cavity to detect small polyps or submucosal fibroids. Therefore, if you are looking for convenient imaging to detect fibroids, polyps, and/or adenomyosis all at once, an SIS trumps a TVUS. (Note: We call it an S-I-S. So when you request it, you can just say the letters.)

However, for patients with multiple large fibroids, sometimes an SIS is impractical because the bulky fibroids make it difficult to fill the uterus with saline. In this situation, your doctor may recommend a different imaging option.

Question 4: How can I find out if I have endometrial cancer or precancer?

If your doctor is concerned about precancer or cancer, they may offer you a *blind endometrial biopsy*. During this type of biopsy, your feet are put in stirrups, and a speculum (the device we use to see your cervix during a Pap smear) is inserted into your vagina. In other words, the initial setup is just like that for a Pap smear. Then, a slender, flexible catheter is inserted into your uterus to sample a small amount of endometrium (see figure 10). That tissue is sent to a lab, where it is checked for cancerous or precancerous cells. As the name implies, the procedure is done "blindly," meaning that after the catheter is inserted into the uterus, the sample is taken from whichever part of the endometrium that it happens to randomly come in contact with. If the precancer or cancer only occupies a small part of the uterus, this technique may miss it.

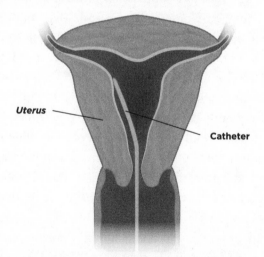

Uterus

Catheter

Figure 10. Blind endometrial biopsy

If cost and availability are not an issue for you, instead of relying on a blind endometrial biopsy, I recommend that you request that your endometrial biopsy be done in conjunction with an *office hysteroscopy* (his-TER-oh-scop-ee). During your office hysteroscopy, which is performed in your ob-gyn's clinic on a regular exam table, you'll be awake as a thin, lighted camera is inserted into your uterus through the vagina. This camera gives your doctor a real-time color video of the inside of your cervix and uterus. If your doctor sees an abnormality during the hysteroscopy, they can make sure they biopsy that part of the endometrium. This increases the odds that the tissue sent to a lab will give you an accurate diagnosis. (Of note, a hysteroscopy will also allow your doctor to visualize and remove uterine or cervical polyps and submucosal fibroids.)

Whether it's done blindly or with hysteroscopy, an office endometrial biopsy can cause quite a bit of cramping, but it usually resolves quickly after the procedure is over. If you don't have a medical reason not to take NSAIDs, consider taking a dose before your appointment to decrease the amount of discomfort you'll experience. Alternatively, your doctor may recommend that you take a different pain medication before your procedure.

If your doctor doesn't offer office hysteroscopy, you can proceed with the blind endometrial biopsy if that's what they recommend. But if the blind biopsy is normal and your bleeding persists in spite of treatment (e.g., with birth control pills), ask your doctor if they think you need further evaluation.

To be clear, I'm not saying that a TVUS mentioned in question 3 or the blind endometrial biopsy discussed in this question will miss every growth, but if an SIS or office hysteroscopy is an option for you, I recommend that you start with that.

Question 5: My doctor confirmed that I have one of those growths. What are some treatment options I should ask about?

See chapter 10 for more information about the birth control options mentioned in this answer.

Some potential treatment options for fibroids,
adenomyosis, polyps, and endometrial cancer/
precancer

Fibroids. See the fibroid spotlight on pages 196–206 for more information.

Adenomyosis. Once medications are stopped — for example, when you want to get pregnant — symptoms usually return within six months. Removal of the uterus is the only guaranteed way to get rid of adenomyosis prior to menopause. Symptoms usually resolve after menopause.

• Treatment options for women not finished having kids:
  ○ **Hormonal birth control.** My top recommendation is a 52 mg levonorgestrel-releasing IUD such as Mirena. But you can also try other options, including continuous birth control (pills, patches, or rings), the birth control shot, or the arm implant.
  ○ **NSAIDs.** To decrease menstrual flow, start the med on the first day of bleeding and continue for four or five days or until menstruation ceases. (Example: Ibuprofen 600 mg once per day.) If you have pain with your bleeding, you should start the NSAID a couple of days before your period is expected to start. On page 171, I discuss NSAID regimens that are more likely to help with period pain; those regimens might also decrease your bleeding.
  ○ **Tranexamic acid.** This is a nonhormonal medication that is only taken during your period. In many patients, it decreases bleeding significantly. Dosing: tranexamic acid 1.3 grams by mouth 3 times daily for up to five days during period (started with onset of heavy menstrual bleeding).
  ○ **GnRH antagonist or GnRH agonist.** People

typically try this if several birth control options and NSAIDs don't work. Elagolix, for example, is an oral GnRH antagonist that can be used for up to twenty-four months. See page 172 for more information about GnRH antagonists and agonists.

○ **Uterus-sparing resection of adenomyosis.** An investigational procedure may occasionally be offered if a woman with extensive adenomyosis is actively pursuing pregnancy. The uterus-sparing resection of adenomyosis is when a surgeon cuts the adenomyosis out of a woman's uterus. If you get pregnant after this procedure, you have an increased risk of uterine rupture between 12 and 35 weeks of gestation (meaning the uterine scar from the surgery opens up during your pregnancy) and abnormal placental attachment (which is when the baby's placenta doesn't attach to the uterine wall in a normal manner).

• Treatment options for women finished having kids:

○ **Uterine artery embolization.** This is when tiny particles are injected into the blood vessels that lead to the uterus. These particles block blood flow and therefore starve the adenomyosis tissue, causing shrinkage and decreasing symptoms.

○ **Hysterectomy.** This is surgical removal of the uterus. Since adenomyosis is confined to the uterus, you don't need to remove your ovaries.

Polyps (cervical or endometrial). If you have a polyp that is causing heavy or irregular bleeding, it needs to be removed and evaluated under a microscope to make sure it isn't cancerous or precancerous.

Some cervical polyps can be easily removed in the clinic. For this procedure, after inserting a vaginal speculum, your healthcare practitioner will use polyp forceps to grasp the base of the polyp and gently twist it. It's quick and painless. I've never had a patient complain of discomfort with an in-office cervical polyp removal.

If you have polyps inside your uterus or if the practitioner cannot see the base of your cervical polyp during the speculum exam, you should have a hysteroscopy to remove it under direct visualization. If you need hysteroscopy for the removal, ask if it can be done in the clinic instead of the operating room. Why? An in-office procedure can quickly remove your polyp while saving you the hassle associated with going to the operating room.

Endometrial cancer or precancer. Whether you're dealing with cancer or precancer, always, always, always make sure you follow up exactly as instructed. Treatment may include hormonal medication, surgery, radiation, and/or chemotherapy.

If you are diagnosed with precancer or cancer, I recommend that you ask to be referred to a gynecologic oncologist (a doctor who specializes in caring for patients with cancers of the female reproductive tract). If you have cancer, the oncologist should assume your care. For precancer, the oncologist may take over your care or they may work closely with your ob-gyn to ensure that you have the best possible treatment plan.

DR. NITA'S NOTE
Uterine Fibroid Spotlight

What are fibroids? Fibroids, which are also known as leiomyomas (lie-oh-my-OH-mas) or myomas, are noncancerous growths in the muscular wall of the uterus.

Why do people get fibroids? We don't know what

causes them, but they seem to respond to the female hormones estrogen and progesterone. Some factors that increase your risk of fibroids include high blood pressure, obesity, or having a family history of them.

How common are they? Fibroids are the most common pelvic tumor in females. They're estimated to occur in up to 80 percent of women by menopause. They usually occur between the ages of thirty and forty, but they can happen at any age. Compared with white women, Black women are two to three times more likely to have fibroids.

What are the symptoms? Some people don't have any symptoms. But those who do might notice heavy or irregular periods, fatigue due to anemia, abdominal discomfort or fullness, lower back pain, painful periods, painful sex, miscarriages, infertility, frequent urination or trouble emptying their bladder, or bowel symptoms such as constipation. Black women tend to have bigger fibroids, more severe symptoms, and a higher chance of getting fibroids at an early age. When reproductive hormone levels go down and periods stop after menopause, most, but not all, patients have shrinkage of fibroids.

How can I prevent more fibroids?

- Ask your doctor to check your vitamin D level. Research suggests that vitamin D deficiency or insufficiency, which is more common in African Americans, may be linked to fibroid risk.
- Watch your diet. Eat less beef and other red meat and more green vegetables and fruit (especially citrus fruits).
- Exercise. Activity may decrease your risk of developing fibroids.
- Take it easy on the alcohol. Consuming alcohol, especially beer, increases your risk of developing fibroids.

How can my fibroids be treated? Some people without symptoms choose not to do anything. If you're in this camp, your practitioner might recommend a yearly evaluation (which may include an ultrasound) to monitor the growth of the fibroid(s).

Surgery and medication are the two primary treatment paths for people with symptoms.

Medications to Help with Bleeding

If your bleeding is so heavy that you're severely anemic, your doctor might recommend surgery instead of medication, or you may need a blood transfusion or an intravenous (IV) iron transfusion.

Some women can have very large fibroids that cause the uterus to be up to ten times its normal size. This causes what we call "bulk symptoms." For example, a woman may feel that her uterus is very enlarged, as if she's pregnant. Or she may have related symptoms due to its bulk size, such as increased urination or constipation. Aside from the temporary relief a GnRH agonist/antagonist may provide, medication probably won't improve bulk symptoms. Those bulk symptoms are best addressed by surgery. But if you are trying to decrease bleeding, the following meds might work. However, it's important to remember that these can help symptoms while you are taking them, but they will not "cure" your fibroids. Once you stop the medication, your symptoms are very likely to return, unless you don't stop taking them until you are menopausal (which is when you reach the point in your life when your ovaries stop producing estrogen and menstrual periods permanently stop).

- **Estrogen-and-progestin-containing birth control (pills, patches, and vaginal rings).** Decreases bleeding but does not slow down fibroid growth or reduce fibroid volume

- **Progestin-containing IUD (such as Mirena IUD).** Decreases bleeding more than birth control pills. However, the risk of expulsion (which is when your IUD comes out) is increased, especially if your fibroid is completely or partially submucosal.

- **Tranexamic acid.** This is one of my favorite treatment options in the entire book. It has no effect on fibroid size, but this nonhormonal oral antifibrinolytic agent frequently works wonders for patients when it comes to decreasing bleeding. And instead of a daily pill, you only take it for up to five days a month. Dosing: Tranexamic acid 1.3 g by mouth 3 times daily for up to five days during your period (started with onset of heavy menstrual bleeding).

- **GnRH antagonist.** This is a new, exciting option that you should know about! This medication, which is available in an oral form, reduces heavy bleeding and fibroid volume. It works by putting your body in what you can think of as "temporary menopause," which will decrease your estrogen levels. But the menopausal side effects (such as hot flashes and bone loss) can be alleviated by taking "add back" therapy, which is a very low dose of estrogen and progestin. Oriahnn, a GnRH antagonist with estrogen and progestin add back, is currently FDA approved for up to twenty-four months of use to treat heavy menstrual bleeding associated with uterine fibroids. This medication is an excellent option for women who are close to menopause or individuals who need surgery but want to put it off for a while. The downside is that once you stop the medication, your symptoms will return. And it's expensive without insurance coverage.

- **GnRH agonist.** This medication reduces heavy bleeding and significantly reduces fibroid size. It is usually used to (a) shrink fibroids before a surgery so that patients can have a less invasive procedure, (b) stop bleeding to improve anemia before surgery, or (c) serve as transitional therapy for people who are very close to menopause and need their fibroid symptoms to be well-controlled until then. Once you stop taking the GnRH agonist your symptoms will return and the fibroid(s) will grow back to pretreatment levels within three to nine months. Like GnRH antagonists, it works by putting your body into "temporary menopause," which will decrease your estrogen level. Because of the risk of long term decreased estrogen, treatment of fibroids with GnRH agonists is typically limited to three to six months. Unfortunately, it's expensive without insurance coverage.
- **NSAIDs.** Decrease heavy bleeding and pain but less effectively than estrogen-and-progestin birth control, the progestin-containing IUD, or tranexamic acid.
- **Aromatase inhibitors.** Limited evidence demonstrates reduction in bleeding and fibroid size. More research is needed.
- **Natural therapies (vitamin D and epigallocatechin gallate).** May inhibit fibroid growth. More research is needed.

I do not recommend the use of herbal supplements such as black cohosh or Chinese herbal medicine because there aren't large, well-designed studies to prove that these options are safe and effective when it comes to helping you with your fibroid symptoms.

Procedures/Surgery

I know this is a lot of info, but stick with me. This is important! If you want a surgery that will allow you to keep your uterus so you can have kids in the future, ask questions 1 through 6 below. If you don't want more kids in the future, ask questions 1, 5, and 6.

1. *Do I need an endometrial biopsy before the surgery to rule out endometrial cancer?* Fibroids are almost always not cancerous, but if you are having irregular bleeding, your surgeon needs to be confident that there isn't an underlying endometrial precancer or cancer.

2. *How many fibroids do I have, and how big are they?* You can have one fibroid or a lot of them. And they can be the size of a pea or as large as a watermelon. Sometimes the person who interprets your imaging report won't give an exact number. Instead, they will say that you have "multiple fibroids." And if you have a lot of them, they may measure the smallest one and the largest ones to give a range.

3. *Are they submucosal, intramural, or subserosal?* (See pages 188–89 in this chapter if you need to brush up on these terms.) You don't actually have to use the medical terms when asking this question. Just say, "Are they protruding into my cavity, in the wall of the uterus, or on the outer surface?" Many women have a combination of these different types.

4. (If they are submucosal) *Are they type 0, type 1, or type 2?* Your doctor may be surprised that you know to ask this. As shown in figure 11, the International Federation of Gynecology and Obstetrics (FIGO) has a fibroid subclassification system that organizes fibroids

(depicted by the numbered circles) according to their location in the uterus. Types 0, 1, and 2 are completely or partially submucosal; types 3 and 4 are intramural; types 5, 6, and 7 are subserosal; and type 8 is considered "other" (for example, cervical fibroids). Type 0, type 1, and some type 2 fibroids can be removed vaginally. That means no cuts on your abdomen.

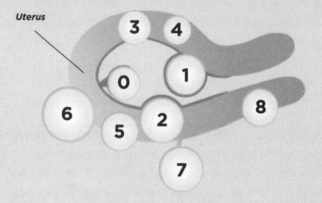

Figure 11. FIGO fibroid subclassification system

5. *Based on the number, size, and location of my fibroids, which treatment options do you offer?* This is an important question. People don't realize that this answer is likely to be very different from the answer to the next question.

6. *Based on the number, size, and location of my fibroids, what are all my treatment options?* Most doctors don't perform or have access to every fibroid procedure/ surgery under the sun. That doesn't make them bad doctors. But before you decide on a treatment plan, you should consider all your options. You might decide that you'd rather have a more invasive procedure with your Dr. Right than a less invasive procedure with a

doctor you don't know. Or your insurance might cover only certain procedures, although you can always call your insurance company to advocate for yourself and request the procedure you want. The point is that you deserve to know all your options before your surgery.

Currently available procedure options if future pregnancy is desired

Do not, I repeat, *do not* let someone convince you to get a hysterectomy for noncancerous fibroids if you want kids in the future. Unless you are in an emergent situation (read: bleeding to death and you need a hysterectomy to save your life or you're dealing with a different, equally serious matter), no one should tell you that a hysterectomy is your only option for noncancerous fibroids.

If you wish to carry a pregnancy in the future, you should have a myomectomy (fibroid removal surgery). Recurrence of fibroids after myomectomy increases over time and approaches 25 percent at forty months. Therefore, you may need another surgery in the future.

- **Hysteroscopic myomectomy.** Decreases bleeding. A small camera is inserted into your uterus and the fibroid is removed. This is a great option for FIGO type 0, FIGO type 1, and some FIGO type 2 submucosal fibroids. If you have fibroids that can be removed with this procedure, this is the surgery you want! You don't have any cuts on your abdomen. You go home the day of the surgery, and recovery is usually a breeze.
- **Laparoscopic (or robotic) myomectomy.** Reduces uterine volume and improves symptoms. Via small

abdominal incisions, a camera is inserted to see your fibroids, and the fibroids are then removed using slender instruments. Recommended for intramural and subserosal fibroids and for patients who have fibroids that are not able to be removed via a hysteroscopic myomectomy.

- **Abdominal myomectomy.** Reduces uterine volume and improves symptoms. A vertical or bikini-cut incision is made on your abdomen, and the fibroids are removed. This invasive type of myomectomy is sometimes recommended when fibroids are large or numerous. But here's some information you should know before you say yes to an abdominal myomectomy, which has a longer recovery time than a laparoscopic myomectomy: If your doctor recommends an abdominal myomectomy, it may be because they don't feel comfortable doing your surgery laparoscopically. That doesn't make them an unqualified or bad doctor. It just means they don't have the expertise needed to perform this particular surgery. Respect their surgical limitations! Under no circumstances should you try to make your doctor perform the procedure laparoscopically if they don't feel comfortable doing so. However, there are a lot of "fibroid gurus" who are willing and able to perform laparoscopic procedures even if fibroids are large or numerous. If your insurance will cover your surgery with a surgeon who has a lot of experience successfully performing laparoscopic myomectomies on women who have large or numerous fibroids, you should strongly consider scheduling a consultation with one of them.

Currently available procedure options if future pregnancy is not desired

- **Endometrial ablation/myolysis.** This procedure reduces your heavy bleeding. Endometrial ablation is the destruction of the endometrium. Myolysis is the destruction of the fibroid. Patient should be premenopausal.
- **Radiofrequency volumetric thermal ablation.** Minimally invasive procedure that uses radiofrequency to reduce fibroid volume and improve symptoms. Impact on fertility requires further investigation.
- **Hysterectomy.** This is when your uterus is removed. This is the only surgery that guarantees you'll never have uterine fibroids again. Removing your uterus will not make you menopausal. However, if you choose to have both of your ovaries removed, you will be in menopause.

    If your fibroids aren't very big, ask if you can have a vaginal hysterectomy. There are no cuts on your abdomen with a vaginal hysterectomy; everything is done through the vagina. If you are told that your uterus is too big to perform the surgery vaginally, ask if you can have a laparoscopic hysterectomy. If your doctor doesn't feel comfortable performing the surgery laparoscopically, respect their surgical limitations. Get a second opinion from a doctor who does a lot of laparoscopic hysterectomies.

    If you have a hysterectomy, ask your doctor to remove your cervix. Removing it eliminates the possibility of cervical cancer or cervical fibroids in the future.
- **Uterine artery embolization (UAE).** During this minimally invasive procedure that reduces symptoms and decreases fibroid volume, small particles are injected

into the arteries supplying the uterus. This cuts off blood flow to the fibroids, causing the fibroids to shrink. One potential complication is that the particles can also cut off blood flow to your ovaries. If that happens, you could go into menopause sooner than you would have if you hadn't had the surgery. Also, people tend to have a lot of pain for the first few days after this procedure. About one in five women who had UAE later needed another surgery for their fibroids. Impact on fertility requires further investigation.

- **MRI-guided focused ultrasound surgery.** Minimally invasive way to control symptoms and reduce fibroid size. This noninvasive treatment takes place in an MRI machine, which guides the treatment. This is a good option for patients who are not good surgical candidates or who choose to avoid surgery. Impact on fertility requires further investigation.

If the treatment option the doctor recommends is not the one you want, ask them why they think theirs is a better choice. Remember that some procedures are appropriate only for certain types of fibroids. But if there's a procedure that interests you, your doctor should be able to tell you why it's not a good option. Advocate for yourself! And don't hesitate to get more than one opinion.

Question 6: We checked, and my doctor said I don't have a growth. Why else might my periods be heavy or irregular?

Another common reason for periods to be heavy or irregular is that you are not ovulating regularly, which means you don't consistently release an egg from your ovary during your menstrual cycle. Here's why anovulation (not ovulating) can be problematic.

Estrogen and progesterone are the two major hormones produced during your menstrual cycle. Normally, estrogen is the predominant hormone during the first half of your cycle. Then, after you ovulate, which happens about two weeks before your next period, the balance shifts and progesterone becomes the predominant hormone. If you don't ovulate, that shift never happens and your body is left with too much estrogen and not enough progesterone. That's problematic for your endometrium (the inside lining of your uterus that you shed during your period).

Your endometrium relies on increasing and decreasing levels of estrogen and progesterone to know when it's time to grow or shed. When someone has *ovulatory cycles*, the predictable estrogen and progesterone fluctuations make their uterine lining grow all at once, then shed all at once. Bleeding is coordinated and orderly. During an *anovulatory cycle*, the bleeding goes haywire. Different parts of the endometrium grow and shed at different rates. As one area of bleeding begins to heal, another area may begin to slough.

The bleeding associated with anovulation that's due to too much estrogen can present in different ways. For example, some people have a little bleeding here and a little bleeding there. Others go months without a period, then *bam!* They have bleeding so heavy that it seems as though someone has opened a floodgate.

But this issue goes beyond annoying irregular periods. If the constant exposure to estrogen without progesterone goes on for a long time, the excessive levels of estrogen can lead to cancer or precancer of the endometrium.

A hormonal imbalance called polycystic ovarian syndrome (PCOS) is a common cause of this type of anovulatory bleeding. Please see the PCOS spotlight below.

DR. NITA'S NOTE
Polycystic Ovarian Syndrome (PCOS) Spotlight

What is polycystic ovary syndrome (also known as polycystic ovarian syndrome or PCOS)? Women with PCOS have a hormonal imbalance and metabolism problems that may affect their overall health and appearance.

Why do people get PCOS? The exact causes aren't known at this time, but higher than normal levels of a male hormone called androgens play an important part.

How common is it? It is one of the most common endocrine disorders found in women. Between 5 and 10 percent of American women who are of childbearing age have it.

What are some things I might notice if I have PCOS? Some people don't have any symptoms. People who do might notice one or more of these issues:

- **Irregular periods.** These can be periods that are absent, heavy, too frequent, not frequent enough, or unpredictable.
- **Hirsutism.** This is when a female has an excessive amount of hair growing on her face (upper lip, chin, neck, sideburn area), chest, abdomen, or upper thighs. Hirsutism affects more than 70 percent of women with PCOS.
- **Acne.** Severe acne or acne that happens after adolescence and doesn't respond to typical treatments is common. In addition to facial acne, up to 50 percent

of women with PCOS have acne that involves the chest, upper back, and neck.

- **Obesity.** Up to 80 percent of women with PCOS are obese.
- **Hair loss.** This may involve thinning of scalp hair or male pattern baldness.
- **Acanthosis nigricans.** These are patches of thick, velvety, darkened skin in body folds and creases, like underneath the breasts, the back of the neck, armpits, or groin. Diabetes and obesity are the most common medical disorders linked with acanthosis nigricans.
- **Infertility.** PCOS is one of the most common causes of infertility.

Note: Don't jump to conclusions and self-diagnose. For instance, some people come from families that tend to have more body hair because of genetic reasons, not because they have PCOS. And there are lots of possible reasons for irregular periods.

How is it diagnosed? There are different ways to diagnose it, but many doctors will diagnose a patient with PCOS if they confirm that another condition that can mimic PCOS isn't causing the patient's symptoms (e.g., a thyroid problem) *and* the patient meets at least two of these three criteria:

- **Anovulation or not ovulating frequently.** This shows up as irregular periods.
- **Signs that you have high levels of male hormones (androgens).** We can base this on blood tests that show a high androgen level or symptoms that are caused by high androgens like hirsutism, acne, or male-pattern

baldness. (If labs are drawn, androgen levels should not be checked when women are on certain medications, including estrogen-containing birth control pills, which can impact androgen levels.)

- **Polycystic ovaries on ultrasound.** An ultrasound may show multiple small cysts.

How can my PCOS be treated? Your treatment should be tailored to your symptoms, health problems, and fertility desires. Common symptoms and medical issues can be treated with the options listed below.

Diet and Exercise

Maintaining a healthy weight and exercising regularly are recommended for all women with PCOS. If you are overweight or obese, losing 5 to 10 percent of your weight (e.g., going from 200 pounds to 190 or 180 pounds) may improve ovulation, pregnancy rates, and overall health. Since weight loss can result in a decrease in serum androgen concentrations, in some instances people will also see improvements in acne and hirsutism. For severely obese women who are unable to lose weight with diet and exercise alone, weight-loss surgery may be appropriate.

Medications and Treatments for Common PCOS Complaints

Utilizing medications and treatments specifically designed to help with hirsutism, acne, infertility, or hair loss is optional, but if a person with PCOS is not ovulating regularly, chronic anovulation must be addressed to prevent endometrial cancer and precancer.

Irregular periods (and cancer/precancer prevention)

If you desire hormonal birth control:

- Estrogen-and-progestin-containing pills, patches, or birth control rings will balance out your estrogen and progesterone levels. The steady presence of progesterone in your birth control will protect your endometrium from cancer. Additionally, hormonal birth control may regulate your menstrual period.

- If you can't use estrogen or you choose not to, a progestin-containing IUD or progestin-only birth control pills are also excellent options.

If you do not desire birth control, but you're still OK with hormones:

- Oral progestin (example: Provera 10 mg for 12 to 14 days every one to two months). This is also a great option to reduce the risk of endometrial cancer.

If you do not wish to use hormones:

- Metformin (an antidiabetic medication). This medication restores ovulatory periods in approximately 30 to 50 percent of women with PCOS. Compared to the hormonal options above, metformin's ability to prevent precancer or cancer of the endometrium is less well established. Therefore, some experts consider metformin to be a less desirable option.

Hirsutism

This list of options is not all-inclusive.

- Estrogen-and-progestin-containing birth control pills are considered first-line therapy. Higher doses of ethinyl estradiol (30 or 35 mcg) are needed in some women for optimal suppression of androgens for management of hirsutism. Although transdermal or vaginal ring preparations are potential options, they have not been well studied for the management of hirsutism.

- An antiandrogen medication (such as spironolactone) is sometimes prescribed, along with the birth control. Alternatively, the antiandrogen can be taken alone. But you should not get pregnant while taking spironolactone; it can prevent development of normal external genitalia in a male fetus.

- Shaving, waxing, hair removal creams, electrolysis, or laser therapy. Research shows that these will not cause hair to grow faster. There is also a topical drug called eflornithine hydrochloride that inhibits hair growth.

Acne

- Estrogen-and-progestin-containing birth control (pills, patches, or the birth control ring).
- Topical acne medication or the antiandrogen spironolactone may also help.
- Acne related to PCOS can be very stubborn. If you are struggling to find something that works, ask for a dermatology referral.

Infertility

If weight loss doesn't cause you to start ovulating again, oral or injected fertility medication, in vitro fertilization, or other fertility treatments may be recommended. See chapter 15 for more information.

Scalp hair loss

Ask for a dermatology referral to discuss treatments to encourage hair growth and prevent further loss.

Emotional health
See a therapist if needed. Research shows that people who have to manage chronic issues like PCOS have a higher incidence of depression and anxiety.

If I have PCOS, is there anything else I need to speak to my doctor about? Yes. People with PCOS have an increased incidence of certain health conditions, including the following:

- **High blood pressure.** Compared to women without PCOS who are the same age, women with PCOS have a higher chance of high blood pressure, the leading cause of stroke and heart disease.
- **Unhealthy cholesterol.** You're more likely to have a lower level of protective "good cholesterol" (HDL) and a higher level of problematic "bad cholesterol" (LDL). That raises your risk of heart disease and stroke.
- **Diabetes.** More than half of women with PCOS will develop prediabetes or diabetes before the age of forty.
- **Sleep apnea.** With sleep apnea, you have repeated stops in breathing that interrupt your sleep. Sleep apnea raises your risk of heart disease and diabetes, and the sleep interruptions can leave you feeling tired all the time.

Researchers do not know if PCOS causes some of these problems, if these problems cause PCOS, or if there are other conditions that cause PCOS and other health problems.

At the time of your initial diagnosis, ask your doctor to check your blood pressure, and ask them if a fasting lipid profile and two-hour glucose tolerance test (OGTT) are appropriate. The reason you want an OGTT is because a fasting blood glucose is often normal even when prediabetes or diabetes is present. The OGTT, which checks your blood sugar levels before and two hours after you drink a special sweet drink, really puts your body to the test and tells the doctor how your body processes sugar. So it's a great way to diagnose prediabetes and/or diabetes in patients with PCOS. But if an OGTT is not possible, get whichever diabetes test is most convenient for you. Also, let your doctor know if you snore. If you do, they may order a sleep study, which is a noninvasive exam that allows doctors to monitor you while you sleep to diagnose sleep apnea.

If you aren't found to have these conditions when you are initially diagnosed with PCOS, maintaining a healthy weight will decrease the probability that you'll develop these health issues in the future. But regardless of your weight, you should have routine check-ups and lab tests to ensure that these conditions are detected and treated early if they do arise.

Question 7: Aside from a growth and ovulation problems, what's another possible cause of heavy/irregular bleeding that I should look out for?

If you meet the criteria for scenarios 1, 2, or 3 described below, your doctor should check your medical history and run some basic labs to ensure that you don't have a bleeding disorder.

Scenario 1. Have you had heavy menstrual bleeding since your first menstrual period?

Scenario 2. Have you had *one* of the following conditions?

- Postpartum hemorrhage. This is when you have very heavy bleeding after delivering a baby.
- Surgery-related bleeding. If you've ever had surgery and your doctor told you that you bled more than they expected.
- Bleeding associated with dental work. This is when you bleed more than expected during a dental procedure.

Scenario 3. Do you experience *two or more* of the following conditions?

- Bruising one to two times a month
- Nose bleeds one to two times a month
- Frequent gum bleeding
- Family history of bleeding symptoms

If you answered "yes" to scenarios 1, 2, or 3, but your initial lab work doesn't show anything and you are still concerned, schedule an appointment with a hematologist (blood doctor) to determine if a more detailed workup is needed.

Question 8. What are some other possible causes for heavy, irregular periods?

There are a lot of possible additional causes. Here are a few you should definitely know about:

- **Perimenopause.** Hormonal fluctuations around menopause can lead to heavy and/or irregular periods. If this happens to you, check in with your doctor to ensure that you don't need an endometrial biopsy.
- **A Cesarean scar defect (CSD).** This is when your uterine scar doesn't heal correctly. CSDs should be considered in women presenting with spotting after periods, painful periods, pelvic pain, or infertility and

a history of c-section. One reason the spotting happens is because endometrium that should have been expelled during your period gets trapped in the defect then it slowly trickles out after your period is over. Common ways to diagnose a CSD are with a transvaginal ultrasound, SIS, or hysteroscopy. It can be treated with hormones to manage your symptoms or surgery to repair the defect. Unfortunately, many physicians are not familiar with this condition; therefore, women may go a long time without an accurate diagnosis.

- **Medication you are taking.** Tell your doctor about all your medications (including supplements) so they can figure out if a medication is the cause. Some potential culprits include hormonal contraception, blood-thinners, and aspirin. Please don't stop taking meds that are necessary before talking to a doctor.
- **An endometrial lining problem.** Sometimes, the endometrium is not functioning the way it should. One reason this can happen is because of an intrauterine infection that needs to be treated. Another potential cause is endometriosis, which is when tissue similar to the inside lining of the uterus is found outside of the uterus.
- **You have periods that are slightly heavier, just because.** We are all different. Therefore, some people will have heavier periods than others. Even if no underlying abnormality is identified, you may still benefit from many of the medications discussed in this chapter, such as hormonal birth control, NSAIDs, or tranexamic acid. Your doctor may also talk to you about surgical procedures. One option is an endometrial ablation, which is a quick outpatient procedure that destroys or removes most of the lining of the uterus. Eight to twelve weeks after the procedure, most

patients with a successful ablation will have lighter periods. In some cases, the ablation stops menstrual bleeding altogether, but this is usually not the case. However, an ablation may not be appropriate if your abnormal bleeding is caused by anovulation. If you opt for an endometrial ablation, make sure you understand the risks and benefits. Due to the increased risk of miscarriage, pregnancy after an ablation is not recommended, but it is possible to get pregnant after an ablation. Therefore, make sure you use effective birth control.

Question 9. Could my bleeding be due to more than one cause?

Yes! So if your healthcare practitioner finds a cause but your bleeding doesn't get better with treatment, consider the possibility that (a) you need to try a different treatment option or (b) something else is going on in addition to the cause you found.

Question 10: We've talked a lot about adults who bleed too much, but aside from PCOS, what are some other reasons an adult might have a period that's missing in action?

This list is not all-inclusive, but here are some reasons why women who were menstruating and who are not pregnant, breastfeeding, or menopausal stop having periods:

- Severe or prolonged illness, such as kidney failure or inflammatory bowel disease (IBD)
- Low body weight (10 percent or more below normal weight)
- Rapid weight loss
- Eating disorders (such as anorexia nervosa)

- Excessive exercise (including running, ballet dancing, figure skating, gymnastics, etc.)
- Elevated prolactin due to pituitary adenoma
- Primary ovarian insufficiency
- Severe stress
- Hypothyroidism
- Hyperthyroidism
- Intrauterine scarring after a surgical procedure (in rare cases, this happens after a D&C has been performed after a miscarriage)
- Certain medications

Of note, not every cause of missing periods leads to increased estrogen or an increased risk of endometrial cancer or precancer, but even if you don't need endometrial protection it's important that you know why your periods are MIA. Therefore, if your period stops for more than three months without a definite explanation, make sure you check in with a doctor so they can determine what's going on. Your treatment will depend on the cause.

DR. NITA'S NOTE
Advocate for Your Health Like a Pro When Your Periods Are Out of Whack

Here are some questions to ask your doctor:
If you're bleeding too much:

1. *Did you notice anything abnormal during my exam today? If so, what did you notice?* Some issues that can be identified during an exam will not show up on imaging. Therefore, you should always get an exam.
2. *What imaging will you order?* As discussed earlier, I

recommend that you start with an SIS or hysteroscopy (depending on what your doctor is most concerned about). If you are unable to get these tests due to cost or availability, please proceed with whichever option works best for you.

3. *Will you check a CBC (complete blood count)? Will you also order iron tests?* These tests determine whether you have iron-deficiency anemia. I recommend both, but if cost is an issue, you may decide to have only the CBC.

4. *Do I need any additional labs or testing?* For example, in addition to evaluating your period issues, your doctor may also need to perform a Pap smear.

5. *Do I need an endometrial biopsy?* Based on risk factors such as your age, weight, and the presence (or absence) of PCOS, your doctor will determine whether you need an endometrial biopsy to rule out cancer or precancer.

6. *How much iron should I take?* (Unless they checked your blood for anemia while you were in the clinic, this advice may change once your labs return.) In addition to your iron pill(s), add iron-rich foods to your diet (do a Google search for the best ones). If you cannot tolerate oral iron or if you are noncompliant with the recommendation to take it, IV iron may be recommended. Iron pills frequently cause constipation, so use a stool softener or fiber supplement as needed. Eating certain foods (such as whole grains) can also help with constipation.

7. *What can I do to help my bleeding while we are doing the workup?* If your bleeding becomes too heavy or you start to experience severe symptoms (such as feeling faint), you should contact your doctor or go to the nearest emergency room.

If your period stops for three or more months without a definite explanation:

1. *Could any of my medications be the cause?* Make sure you bring a complete list of medications (including supplements) so your practitioner can review them.
2. *Do we need to order labs/imaging?* Understand what's being ordered and why they are ordering it.
3. *Do I need an endometrial biopsy?* Based on risk factors such as your age, weight, and the presence (or absence) of PCOS, your doctor will determine if you need an endometrial biopsy to rule out cancer or precancer.
4. *Would any lifestyle changes be helpful?* For example, excessive exercise can cause anovulation.

Tips for your follow-up appointment (assuming you didn't get the diagnosis the first appointment):

- When you arrive for your follow-up appointment, be ready to ask questions! Some people only focus on what their diagnosis is, but it's also nice to know what was ruled out during your workup.
- Once you have a diagnosis, make sure you understand *all* your treatment options, and ensure you understand the risks and benefits of each one. See the questions at the end of chapter 6 (page 132) for advice on what to ask if your appointment is coming to an end and you have no clue what your doctor is talking about.
- If you are dealing with periods that are irregular or totally absent and your treatment plan doesn't involve hormones, ask if you need hormonal medication for endometrial protection.

Chapter 10

Make Your Birth Control Multitask
Birth Control Cheat Sheet

"This is the worst birth control on the planet. It ruined my life." — said by a thirty-two-year-old patient who was trying to get pregnant after taking a Depo-Provera shot without knowing that it can take up to eighteen months to resume ovulation after stopping.

"This is the best birth control in the world. It gave me back my life." — said by a different thirty-two-year-old patient who had been suffering from endometriosis pain until she started taking Depo-Provera.

That's the thing about birth control: It's not one-size-fits-all. Like every other medication on the planet, birth control comes with risks and benefits. So if you are one of the 99 percent of sexually experienced women who will use some form of birth control in their lifetime, here are the basics when it comes to understanding what each option has to offer.

BIRTH CONTROL CRASH COURSE
What You Need to Know to Patient Like a Pro

Question 1: Which types of birth control are 100 percent effective when it comes to preventing pregnancy?

Question 2: I have 0 percent interest in being abstinent or celibate. How effective are some other commonly used options when it comes to preventing pregnancy?

Question 3: You're saying that some of the reversible birth control options are as effective as a vasectomy or female sterilization?

Question 4: I'm not interested in a LARC. What are some facts I should know about the other hormonal options?

Question 5: Which types of birth control are frequently used to help with heavy periods and period cramps?

Question 6: Which types of birth control are your top picks for help with acne, facial hair from PCOS, ovarian cyst prevention, or menstrual migraines?

Question 7: What will hormonal birth control do to my cancer risks?

Question 8: Will using hormonal birth control make it hard to get pregnant after I stop?

Question 9: What are some common side effects of birth control?

Question 10: Which type of birth control is the best?

Question 1: Which types of birth control are 100 percent effective when it comes to preventing pregnancy?

Abstinence and celibacy. That's it. Absolutely, positively nothing else works 100 percent of the time.[1] I'm stressing this because a lot of patients are surprised when I tell them that even tubal ligations aren't 100 percent guaranteed to work.

Question 2: I have 0 percent interest in being abstinent or celibate. How effective are some other commonly used options when it comes to preventing pregnancy?

The table below summarizes the options, and the methods in bold are discussed in more detail after the table. For a list of birth control contraindications, see appendix B (page 385).

Table 6. Effectiveness of Common Birth Control Methods

Birth control	Risk of pregnancy*
Abstinence or celibacy	0 out of 100
Male sterilization (vasectomy, aka "getting snipped")	< 1 out of 100
Female sterilization (aka "getting your tubes tied," "a tubal")	< 1 out of 100
Progestin arm implant	< 1 out of 100
Progestin intrauterine device (IUD)	< 1 out of 100
Copper IUD	< 1 out of 100
Depo-Provera shot ("the birth control shot")	6 out of 100
Estrogen-and-progestin-containing birth control pills	9 out of 100
Progestin-only birth control pills	9 out of 100
Birth control patch	9 out of 100
Vaginal birth control ring	9 out of 100
Diaphragm (when used with a spermicide)	12 out of 100
Male condoms (aka external condoms)	13 out of 100

Table 6. Effectiveness of Common Birth Control Methods
(continued)

Birth control	Risk of pregnancy*
Phexxi (nonhormonal vaginal pH regulator gel)	14 out of 100
Female condoms (aka internal condoms)	21 out of 100
Withdrawal method (pulling out before ejaculation)	22 out of 100
Sponge (a round device that contains spermicide and covers the cervix to keep sperm from entering the uterus)	14 out of 100 if never had a baby; 24 out of 100 if had a baby
Fertility awareness–based methods	2 to 24 out of 100
Cervical cap (a small plastic cap that covers the cervix to keep sperm from entering the uterus and is most effective when used with a spermicide)	16 out of 100 if never had a baby; 32 out of 100 if had a baby
Spermicide	28 out of 100
Lactational amenorrhea	Varies

*   The number of women out of every hundred who will get pregnant within
the first year of typical use of each method.

Female sterilization

Doctors can use different surgical techniques to perform a tubal (short for "tubal sterilization"). While all tubals are highly effective, when you compare the different options, a *salpingectomy* (sal-pin-JEK-tuh-me), which is the complete removal of both fallopian tubes, is the most effective option (see figure 12). Examples of other techniques that have a slightly higher failure rate include cauterizing (burning) the fallopian tubes, tying and cutting them, or cinching them with a band.

The possibility of a uterine pregnancy after salpingectomy is extremely low; one thorough review of research found only four documented pregnancies after this procedure.[2] Plus, since current research shows that many ovarian cancers actually originate in the fallopian tubes, completely removing your tubes substantially reduces your risk of ovarian cancer in the future.

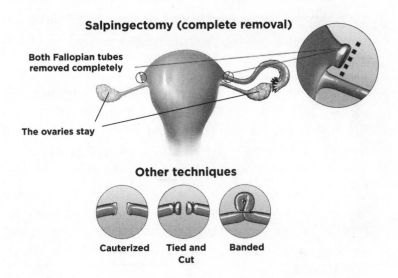

Salpingectomy (complete removal)

Both Fallopian tubes removed completely

The ovaries stay

Other techniques

Cauterized   **Tied and Cut**   **Banded**

Figure 12. Salpingectomy and other techniques for tubals

Phexxi

When semen enters the vagina, it increases the vagina's pH level from its typical acidic range of 3.5 to 4.5 to a range of 6.5 to 7.2. The increased pH allows sperm to swim up the reproductive canal, which is how it reaches an egg to cause pregnancy. When inserted into the vagina, Phexxi, which requires a prescription, maintains a normal vaginal pH in the 3.5 to 4.5 range. This lowers sperm mobility and therefore decreases the chance that sperm will reach the egg. Phexxi was approved for contraceptive use in 2020. Therefore, the failure rate is based on a limited number of studies.

Fertility-awareness based methods

This is when you identify the fertile days of your menstrual cycle by monitoring fertility signs like the consistency of your cervical mucus or your basal body temperature. When you are fertile, you either avoid sex or use a barrier method. Since there are lots of ways of tracking your fertility and some of those ways are more reliable than others, the failure rate can vary a lot.

Spermicides

Most spermicides rely on a chemical called nonoxynol-9 (N-9). Whether they have N-9 or not, spermicides do not protect against any sexually transmitted infections. In fact, N-9 may increase the risk of getting HIV from an infected partner if used many times per day. Therefore, while spermicides may help prevent pregnancy, they may increase your risk of getting an STI if you're exposed. Additionally, spermicides can disrupt the balance between good and bad bacteria in the vagina, and they can also increase the risk of urinary tract infections in some women.

Lactational amenorrhea

For women who have recently had a baby and are breastfeeding, the lactational amenorrhea method (LAM) can be used as birth control when these three conditions are met: (1) less than six months have passed since the baby was delivered; (2) amenorrhea, meaning no menstrual periods have occurred since the baby was delivered; and (3) exclusive, frequent breastfeeding, with the time between feedings no longer than four hours during the day or six hours at night. LAM is a temporary method of birth control, and another birth control method must be used when any of the three conditions are not met. When used correctly, it is very effective contraception, but failure rates vary because many women use this method as birth control without meeting all the criteria.

Question 3: You're saying that some of the reversible birth control options are as effective as a vasectomy or female sterilization?

Yes! They're called long-acting reversible contraceptives (LARCs). The implant, progestin-containing IUD, and copper IUD are each more than 99 percent effective.

I love LARCs because if there is even a 0.00001 percent chance that you'll want kids in the future, you can have the best of both worlds: very effective birth control and the possibility of a future pregnancy. Plus, since they last for several years without any maintenance required, they're super convenient. And the hormonal ones can help with some period complaints.

Here's a little more info about them.

Progestin-containing arm implant

- **What it is:** A small rod (about the size of a matchstick) that releases progestin. It is inserted under the skin of a woman's upper arm.
- **Brand name:** Nexplanon
- **Risk of pregnancy:** Less than 1 in 100
- **Pros:**
  - FDA approved for three years (some studies suggest that it is effective for up to 5 years)
  - Removable whenever you are ready, with no long-term effects on fertility
  - Does not contain estrogen

- **Cons:**
  - Must be inserted and removed by a healthcare practitioner
  - No protection against sexually transmitted infections (STIs)
  - Small risk of pain or infection at the insertion site; risk of difficult removal if it's inserted too deep
- **Major complaint:** A common reason people ask for the implant to be removed is persistent irregular bleeding.

Progestin-containing IUD

- **What it is:** A small progestin-containing T-shaped device that is inserted into the uterus
- **Brand names:** Mirena (52 mg of a progestin called levonorgestrel), Liletta (52 mg of levonorgestrel), Kyleena (19.5 mg of levonorgestrel), and Skyla (13.5 mg of levonorgestrel)
- **Risk of pregnancy:** Less than 1 in 100
- **Pros:**
  - Currently FDA approved for 3 to 7 years (Mirena: 7 years, Liletta: 6 years, Kyleena: 5 years, Skyla: 3 years)
  - Removable whenever you are ready, with no long-term effects on fertility
  - Does not contain estrogen
- **Cons:**
  - Must be inserted and removed by a healthcare practitioner
  - No protection against sexually transmitted infections (STIs)
  - Small risk of uterine perforation during the IUD insertion, and some women have discomfort during insertion

- **Major complaint:** People frequently complain of irregular vaginal spotting for the first three to six months of use. But after that, periods frequently become less crampy and lighter. Some women even stop having periods because the progestin makes the inside lining of the uterus very thin. Mirena and Liletta are more likely to stop your periods because they contain more progestin than the other options.

Copper IUD

- **What it is:** A small nonhormonal T-shaped device that is inserted into the uterus
- **Brand name:** Paragard
- **Risk of pregnancy:** Less than 1 in 100
- **Pros:**
  - FDA approved for 10 years (but several studies say it provides protection for 12 years)
  - Removable whenever you are ready, with no long-term effects on fertility
  - No hormones
- **Cons:**
  - Must be inserted and removed by a healthcare practitioner
  - No protection against sexually transmitted infections (STIs)
  - Small risk of uterine perforation during the IUD insertion, and some women have discomfort during insertion
- **Major complaint:** A common reason people ask for the copper IUD to be removed is that their periods are persistently heavier and crampier. But these symptoms improve within twelve months for many women.

Question 4: I'm not interested in a LARC. What are some facts I should know about the other hormonal options?

Hormonal birth control comes in two forms. One type contains estrogen and progestin. The second type only contains progestin. (Progestin is a form of progesterone, the hormone that plays a role in the menstrual cycle.)

Estrogen-and-progestin-containing options

These are known as *combined hormonal contraception* (CHC).

- **Birth control pills.** You will take one of these pills every day. Some brands have twenty-one days of pills with active hormones and seven days of placebo (sugar) pills. Other brands have twenty-four days of active pills and four days of sugar pills. With either option, you typically get your period while taking the sugar pills. (Note: we call them sugar pills, but with some birth control brands they contain something beneficial, like either iron or a low dose of estrogen that will help reduce bleeding, bloating, and other side effects sometimes associated with a hormone-free interval.) To maximize the effectiveness, you should take the active pill at the same time every day.
- **Vaginal birth control ring.** Brand names: Nuva-Ring and Annovera. This is a flexible ring that you put in your vagina, where hormones are slowly absorbed. Typically, you wear the ring inside the vagina for three weeks, followed by one week when you don't; bleeding occurs during the ring-free week. With NuvaRing, your old ring is discarded and a brand-new ring is used every four weeks. With Annovera, the same ring is used for up to one year (thirteen 28-day cycles). After the Annovera ring has been used for several months,

it may become discolored, but this does not mean the ring is less effective or dirty.

Your birth control ring can be left in place while having sex, but if desired you may take the ring out of the vagina for up to two hours (Annovera) or three hours (NuvaRing and its generic brands). However, the rules about removing it are very specific. For example, if Annovera is out of your vagina for more than two hours at one time or at different times that add up to more than two hours over the twenty-one days of continuous use, then you will need to use another form of birth control (such as a male condom) until Annovera has been in your vagina for seven consecutive days.

- **Birth control patch.** This is a small (1.75 square inch) adhesive patch that is worn on the skin in one of several places, such as the shoulder, belly, back, or hip. You typically wear a new patch each week for three weeks and then leave the patch off during week four, which is when you have your period. It can be worn during activities such as bathing, exercising, and swimming.

Depending on how frequently you wish to have a period, combined hormonal contraception can be taken in different regimens:

- **Cyclic.** With this regimen, you have a period once a month.
  - **Pills.** You take the active (estrogen-and-progestin-containing) pills and placebo pills, as described above. As a result, you have a period every twenty-one or twenty-four days, depending on how many sugar pills you have in your pack. (Exception: Some people won't have a period during the sugar pills.

This is more common with lower dose estrogen-and-progestin containing birth control pills because the low estrogen in the pill — relative to the much larger progestin doses — causes the uterine lining to be so thin that there's nothing to shed during the placebo pills. Not having a period during the placebo week is perfectly safe, but if this bothers you, ask your clinician to increase the estrogen dosage in the pill.)

- ○ **Vaginal ring.** As described above, the ring is worn inside the vagina for twenty-one days and then removed for seven days. During those seven days, you will have your menstrual period. Then after a week, you insert a new NuvaRing or you reinsert your Annovera.

- ○ **Patch.** A new patch is worn for a week at a time for three weeks in a row. During the fourth week, a patch is not worn, and you will have your period.

- **Extended cycle.** With this regimen, you don't stop the active hormones until you are ready to have a period — for example, you may wish to have a period every three months.

  - ○ **Pills.** Take an active pill every day for three months. Take the sugar pills for seven days at the completion of those three months.

  - ○ **Vaginal ring.** Remove the NuvaRing and insert a new one immediately every twenty-one days. Leave the ring out for one week every three months.

  - ○ **Patch.** Apply a new patch every seven days. Have a patch-free week every three months.

- **Continuous dosing.** With this regimen, you don't have a period.

  - ○ **Pills.** Take a pill with active hormones every day. You never take sugar pills.

- ○ **Vaginal ring.** Remove the NuvaRing and insert a new one immediately every twenty-one days. You never have a ring-free week.
- ○ **Patch.** Apply a new patch every week on the same day, without skipping a week.

Progestin-only options

This type of birth control can be used if someone cannot (or does not want to) use estrogen. In addition to the IUDs and implant discussed in question 3, your other progestin-only options include the following:

- **Progestin-only pill (POP).** Unlike traditional birth control pills, the progestin-only pill, also called the mini pill, does not contain estrogen. POPs available in the United States include norethindrone 0.35 mg tablets and drospirenone 4 mg tablets. Norethindrone progestin-only pills need to be taken at the same time every day to prevent pregnancy and decrease the chance of breakthrough bleeding. If you forget to take a norethindrone pill for more than three hours past your usual time, take the pill as soon as you remember and use a backup contraceptive method (e.g., condoms) for at least two days after the late dose. If you miss or forget to take a drospirenone pill, you have twenty-four hours to make up for it without having to add a backup birth control.
- **Birth control shot.** (Brand name: Depo-Provera.) With this option, you will get a shot in a muscle, such as the upper arm or butt, every three months. There is also a version that is given under the skin every three months. An FDA warning states:

Women who use Depo-Provera Contraceptive Injection may lose significant bone mineral density [bone strength]. Bone loss is greater with increasing duration of use and may not be completely reversible. It is unknown if use of Depo-Provera Contraceptive Injection during adolescence or early adulthood, a critical period of bone accretion, will reduce peak bone mass and increase the risk for osteoporotic fracture in later life. Depo-Provera Contraceptive Injection should not be used as a long-term birth control method (i.e., longer than 2 years) unless other birth control methods are considered inadequate.[3]

However, after careful evaluation of the current research, reputable organizations, including the American College of Obstetricians and Gynecologists, state that although the use of the shot is associated with loss of bone mineral density (BMD), evidence suggests that losses in BMD appear to be substantially or fully reversible.[4] Therefore, the effect of Depo on bone strength and potential fracture risk should not prevent practitioners from prescribing the shot or continuing use beyond two years. To promote bone health, Depo-Provera users should have adequate intake of calcium and vitamin D, exercise regularly, and avoid cigarette smoking and excessive alcohol consumption — but this is good advice for all women, regardless of their contraceptive choice.

And just in case you're wondering if it's safe to use birth control to skip periods for months (or even years) at a time, the answer is "Yes!," no matter which of the estrogen-and-progestin-containing or progestin-only hormonal options you choose.

Note: Always make sure you understand the risks and benefits of any option you are considering.

DR. NITA'S NOTE
Emergency Contraception Spotlight

Emergency contraception (EC) can prevent up to approximately 99 percent of pregnancies if taken within five days after intercourse. According to the World Health Organization, "Emergency contraception cannot interrupt an established pregnancy or harm a developing embryo." So, to be clear, emergency contraception is *not* an abortifacient.

Who can use it? Anybody who needs EC to avoid an undesired pregnancy. There are no age limits or medical contraindications to the use of emergency contraception. (Exception: eligibility criteria for general use of IUDs also apply for use of an IUD for EC purposes.)

What are my options? If you find yourself needing it, remember that not all emergency contraception is created equal. And even though you have a few days to use each method, EC should be initiated as soon as possible after unprotected or inadequately protected sex. The sooner you use it, the better it works.

Tier I: The Copper IUD

This is the most reliable type of EC available. To get an IUD (intrauterine device), you must have a negative pregnancy test, understand that there's still some risk of pregnancy, and agree to return to your healthcare practitioner if you discover you're pregnant.

- For effective emergency contraception: insert as soon as possible, but within five days (120 hours) of unprotected sex
- Pregnancy rate in studies: less than 1 percent
- Pros: highly effective at any time in your menstrual cycle, doesn't contain hormones, provides contraception for at least ten years when left in place, and is highly effective regardless of your body mass index (BMI)
- Cons: requires an office visit for a practitioner to insert the IUD, high cost if uninsured, you must call beforehand to ask your clinician if they have an IUD available for insertion (if one needs to be ordered, it may not arrive within your five-day time frame).
- Common side effects: irregular bleeding, heavy periods, and period pain. These side effects usually decrease within a year of having the copper IUD.

Some experts also recommend 52 mg progestin-IUDs for EC, but others, including the American College of Obstetricians and Gynecologists, state that we need more studies before recommending this option. Progestin-IUDs may be more widely accepted as effective emergency contraception after additional studies are completed.

Tier II: Oral Emergency Contraception Medications

There are three options in this tier.

Ulipristal acetate (UPA), sold as Ella

- For effective emergency contraception: take 30 mg as soon as possible, but within five days (120 hours) after unprotected sex
- Pregnancy rate in studies: 1.2–1.8 percent
- Pros: comes in a pill form and is the most effective oral EC

- Cons: requires a prescription, may be less effective if you weigh more than 195 pounds
- Common side effects: suppressed menstruation (may come more than seven days later than expected), abdominal pain, headache, nausea, fatigue

Levonorgestrel (LNG), sold as Plan B

- For effective emergency contraception: take as soon as possible, but within three days (seventy-two hours) after unprotected sex (some experts feel that it can still be effective if taken within five days, but that's an off-label use)
- Pregnancy rate in studies: 2.1–2.6 percent
- Pros: no prescription or ID needed and no age restriction for Plan B One Step
- Cons: may be less effective if you weigh more than 155 pounds
- Common side effects: heavy or prolonged menstrual period, abdominal pain, headache, nausea, fatigue

Yuzpe method

This is when a woman takes everyday estrogen-and-progestin-containing birth control pills as emergency contraception to prevent an unplanned pregnancy before it starts.

- For effective emergency contraception: take as soon as possible, but within five days (120 hours) after unprotected sex. For the initial dose, take 100 to 120 mcg of ethinyl estradiol, plus 0.5 mg to 0.6 mg of levonorgestrel. The same dose is repeated twelve hours after the first dose. The number of pills needed for EC differs for each brand of pill. To find out how many pills you should take for the brand that you have, you can ask a healthcare professional, or you can google "Yuzpe method."

- Pregnancy rate in studies: variable (but higher than the other EC options)
- Pros: accessibility in rural areas or if you're concerned about privacy
- Cons: least effective EC method
- Common side effects: a lot of nausea and vomiting (if needed, you can ask your doctor to prescribe an anti-nausea medication)

Here are answers to some additional questions you might have about emergency contraception:

What if I vomit? We don't have a lot of research to tell us what to do. I recommend taking another dose if you vomit within three hours of taking an oral emergency contraceptive.[5]

Can I rely on my EC for other unprotected sexual encounters during the same menstrual cycle? If you used an oral method, no. If you have an IUD, yes. The copper IUD will remain in place and serve as your birth control.

Can oral EC be used again in the same cycle? Yes, but it's better to use a regular birth control method instead of relying on EC repeatedly. Birth control that is used correctly and consistently is more effective than emergency contraception.

Will emergency contraception protect me from STIs/STDs? No.

Do I need to take a pregnancy test later? If your period doesn't start within three weeks of taking oral emergency contraception, you should take a urine pregnancy test. If you had an IUD inserted, you will probably have irregular bleeding. Therefore, take a urine pregnancy test two to four weeks after placement of the IUD or at any time if you notice pregnancy symptoms.

What if I get pregnant anyway? If this happens, it's because you were pregnant before you used the emergency contraception, the EC failed, or you got pregnant from subsequent sex. Oral EC has not been linked to congenital anomalies or pregnancy complications when pregnancy does occur. But if you had an IUD inserted, it should be removed, if possible. Regardless of the EC method used, pregnancy options and counseling should be provided with linkage to desired care for pregnancy continuation or abortion.

When should I start progestin-containing birth control? After levonorgestrel (LNG) oral EC or the Yuzpe method, you can start or resume any hormonal birth control method right away, but you should also abstain from sex or use a backup method of contraception (such as a condom) for one week. (With the Yuzpe method, start birth control after taking the second dose of pills.) If you took UPA, wait five days to begin or resume any type of hormonal birth control; otherwise, you may decrease the effectiveness of the emergency contraception and the birth control. You also must abstain from sex or use a backup method of contraception (such as a condom) until your next period.

Will emergency contraception impact my ability to get pregnant in the future? No.

Question 5: Which types of birth control are frequently used to help with heavy periods and period cramps?

- Any of the progestin IUDs (*not* the copper IUD)
- Birth control pills

- Birth control ring
- Birth control patch
- Depo-Provera
- Birth control implant

When using birth control that has estrogen and progestin, many patients have better symptom control when they use the extended-cycle or continuous regimens. If you experience irregular vaginal spotting while using the extended or continuous regimen, ask your practitioner if you can stop your pills for three or four days to have a period. Allowing your body to have a short period will frequently cause the annoying unscheduled bleeding to stop. However, to maintain contraceptive benefits, this must be done after twenty-one days of active hormones. Do not use this technique more than once in any four-week cycle.

Regardless of which method you pick, remember that when you start any type of hormonal birth control, it will likely take three to six months for your body to adjust. During that time, it's common to experience irregular bleeding. However, as time progresses, many women have lighter, less crampy periods with the birth control options listed above. For example, you are very likely to have irregular bleeding when you start Depo-Provera. But approximately 50 percent of women will achieve amenorrhea (meaning they will stop having a period) after one year of using it, and over 70 percent will report amenorrhea with longer duration of use. To find the best fit for you, some trial and error may be involved.

In addition to hormonal birth control, there are nonhormonal medication options for heavy periods and period pain. And in some cases, surgery (not medicine) is the appropriate treatment for heavy or painful periods. See chapters 8 and 9 for further details.

Question 6: Which types of birth control are your top picks for help with acne, facial hair from PCOS, ovarian cyst prevention, or menstrual migraines?

- **Acne.** Birth control pills containing estrogen and progestin (you might have the most luck with a pill that has 30 mcg of estrogen and a progestin called drospirenone), the birth control ring, or the birth control patch may help.

- **Hirsutism (facial hair) from PCOS.** My top pick is birth control pills containing estrogen and progestin (you may need a pill with 30 or 35 mcg of estrogen). You can also opt for the vaginal ring or patch, but they have not been well studied for the management of hirsutism.

- **Ovarian cysts.** Hormonal birth control won't make your current cyst(s) go away, but by preventing ovulation they *may* prevent *new* cysts. I typically prescribe a birth control pill containing estrogen and progestin (use a pill with 30 or 35 mcg of estrogen), the birth control patch, or a birth control ring.

- **Menstrual migraines.** These are migraines that happen around the beginning of the menstrual period, usually two days before to three days after the period begins. But people with menstrual migraines may also have migraines at other times during the month.

  If you have migraines with aura (meaning the migraine starts after sensory disturbances like flashes of light or tingling in your hands), I suggest that you stick with nonhormonal treatment options, such as triptans, if possible. If you don't have migraines with aura and you don't have any other contraindications to estrogen, I recommend that you use birth control pills with estrogen and progestin or the vaginal ring continuously.

Question 7: What will hormonal birth control do to my cancer risks?

Using estrogen-and-progestin-containing birth control pills for five years or longer may cut your ovarian cancer risk in half. And that ovarian cancer protection may last up to twenty-five years after you stop taking the pill. On top of that, your risk of endometrial cancer may be cut in half if you take an estrogen-and-progestin-containing pill for at least four years, and this protection lasts for ten years after you stop taking the pill.[6] These birth control pills may also decrease your risk of colorectal cancer.

Using estrogen-and-progestin-containing birth control pills might slightly raise your breast cancer and cervical cancer risks. But your risk goes back to normal about five to ten years after you go off the pill.

We don't have as many studies on the birth control ring or patch, but it is likely that they have the same effects on cancer risks.

We don't have enough research to definitively say how progestin-only birth control impacts breast cancer risk, but it does provide protection from endometrial cancer.

Question 8: Will using hormonal birth control make it hard to get pregnant after I stop?

If you use the Depo-Provera shot, maybe. With all other forms of birth control, no.

Fifty percent of women who discontinue Depo-Provera to become pregnant will conceive within ten months after their last shot, but it can take up to eighteen months to start ovulating again after stopping Depo-Provera. Therefore, although it doesn't permanently impact your fertility, it may take longer to get pregnant after using the birth control shot. With all other forms of hormonal birth control, return to fertility happens quickly, with many women having a menstrual period within 30 days after stopping birth control and almost all women having a menstrual period and return of fertility after ninety days.

However, if you start taking birth control at age twenty-two and stop at age thirty-seven to try to conceive, you will be less fertile at age thirty-seven due to the natural aging process. Or you could have difficulty conceiving because of decreased fertility due to an underlying medical issue (e.g., PCOS). But neither issue has anything to do with the hormonal birth control.

DR. NITA'S NOTE ABOUT FERTILITY
A Woman's Peak Reproductive Years: From Late Teens to Late Twenties

With all the fertility treatment advancements available and women having babies later in life, it's easy to have an "I'll get to it later" attitude when it comes to having kids. However, I want you to remember that you don't know the details of most people's conception journey. Is it possible to have a healthy baby "later in life" without fertility treatments? Yes. (My mom actually had me without fertility assistance after the age of thirty-five.) But don't make assumptions about your future fertility based on what you see going on around you. Sometimes that beautiful baby that you see a forty- or fifty-year-old woman holding is the result of years and years of infertility treatments, or they got pregnant using eggs or embryos (eggs plus sperm) that they froze when they were younger. Or some people use donor eggs (eggs from another person), use surrogates, and so on. Of course, there is nothing wrong with those options, but I don't want you to think that every biological conception comes easily.

Here's the scoop: Fertility decreases gradually throughout life, but starting at age thirty-two the decrease starts to pick up speed, and by thirty-seven the decline is even faster. By the age of forty-five, the probability of pregnancy without fertility assistance is extremely low. But the eggs don't just decrease in number as time progresses, they also decrease in quality. So if you do get pregnant, you also have a higher probability of having a baby with a chromosomal abnormality. Additionally, your chances of experiencing maternal pregnancy-related complications like high blood pressure and diabetes increase with age.

If you aren't ready for babies yet but you are concerned about how aging will affect your fertility, maybe egg or embryo freezing is a good option for you. Frozen eggs and embryos don't continue to age, and they can be stored indefinitely. That means that hypothetically speaking, if a woman freezes her eggs today, in ten or fifteen years they will be as young and healthy as they were when she froze them. But if your insurance company doesn't pay for it, egg and embryo freezing is expensive. And if you do decide to freeze your eggs or embryos, remember that nothing is guaranteed. The only way to be 100 percent certain that you'll conceive is to actually conceive.

Really think about whether you want (more) kids. If your answer is "absolutely not" and you are 100 percent sure, then you're all set. But if there is even a 0.001 percent chance that you think you maybe... might... kinda want biological kids in the future, keep your fertility in mind because even if you look ten years younger than you actually are as an adult, your ovaries will not be deceived (no matter how great your under-eye cream or exercise regimen is).

If you are interested in freezing eggs or embryos, I suggest that you ask your ob-gyn to recommend a reproductive endocrinologist and infertility specialist because not all egg and embryo freezing facilities are created equal! Some are better than others, so choose wisely.

Question 9: What are some common side effects of birth control?

Table 7. Side Effects of Common Birth Control Methods

Birth control	Common side effects
Birth control pills (estrogen-and-progestin and progestin-only)	Headache Nausea Breast tenderness Breakthrough bleeding
Vaginal ring	Headache Breast tenderness Nausea Vaginal discharge Vaginal irritation Breakthrough bleeding
Contraceptive skin patch	Skin irritation Headache Breast tenderness Nausea Breakthrough bleeding

Table 7. Side Effects of Common Birth Control Methods
(continued)

Birth control	Common side effects
Depo-Provera	Weight gain Headache Irregular bleeding (amount usually decreases with each injection)
Implant	Weight gain Irregular bleeding Digestive problems Headaches Breast pain Acne
Progestin IUD	Irregular bleeding Headaches Nausea Breast tenderness Mood changes
Copper IUD	Irregular bleeding Period cramps

The fact that birth control can make headaches go away in some people but can cause headaches in others is a perfect example of how birth control is not one-size-fits-all.

Question 10: Which type of birth control is the best?

There is no one-size-fits-all birth control option. A perfect birth control pill for one woman might be a nauseating, headache-causing, libido-killing mess for another. However, if you are willing to go through some trial and error, it's very likely that you'll find an option that's a good fit for you.

DR. NITA'S NOTE

Advocate for Your Health Like a Pro When You Want Hormonal Birth Control

1. Consider all the major things birth control can do for you (this list is not all-inclusive):
    - Prevent pregnancy
    - Regulate periods
    - Decrease bleeding
    - Lessen period pain
    - Improve acne
    - Lessen PCOS hair growth
    - Help prevent migraines
    - Help prevent ovarian cysts
    - Reduce the chance of some types of cancer
    - Improve PMS/PMDD symptoms (see chapter 7 for more info)
    - Help with hot flashes during the menopause transition (see chapter 14 for more info)
2. Tell your doctor all the issues you'd like your birth control to help with. (Of course, if you only need it to do one thing, that's fine.) For example, you might say, "It's most important for my birth control to decrease my period pain, and I also want something that will help my acne and the migraines I get during my period."
3. Ask which birth control method is the most convenient and effective one if you just want your most important request addressed. In the example I gave, this would mean asking for the options that would conveniently and effectively help your period pain.
4. Ask if any options can address all your requests. Of course, your options will probably be more limited if

your goal is to make your birth control multitask, and there's a chance you may have to prioritize your wish list.

5. Ask about the risks, benefits, and common side effects of the recommended option(s).

6. Once you decide which type of hormonal birth control you want to use, say, "Based on my medical history, is there any reason why it's not safe for me to pick (insert the name of the birth control)?" Hopefully they won't recommend anything that wouldn't be safe, but this question is an extra layer of protection that encourages your practitioner to think about your medical history before writing your prescription. For example, estrogen-containing birth control should not be used in smokers who are thirty-five years old or older. See appendix B for a complete list of contraindications for the different birth control methods.

Chapter 11

Cancer Prevention Is a Big Deal
Cancer Screening Guidelines

People fall behind on their Pap smears and breast cancer screening for many reasons. Here are a few of the most common reasons, along with my tough-love rebuttals.

Patient: I know my body.

My tough-love rebuttal: I can't argue with that statement. Nobody knows your body better than you. That's why doctors need to take your complaints seriously. But does knowing your body also mean that you'd know if there was a nonpalpable early-stage breast cancer hiding deep beneath your skin that can be detected only by routine breast imaging? Would you be able to detect a symptomless cancer or precancer of the cervix without cervical cancer screening? The answer to the first question is nope. And so is the answer to the second one.

Patient: I really want to come in, but I don't want to bring my child(ren) with me, and it's hard to find childcare.

My tough-love rebuttal: I understand that it can be hard to find childcare for a morning or afternoon, but imagine how difficult it would be if you put off the appointment for so long that you ended up being diagnosed with late-stage breast or cervical cancer. Or (God forbid) if you got really sick or passed away, who'd take care of your kids and love them 24/7? Your love for your children is a big reason why you should do everything in your power to get your breasts professionally checked out and get your feet in some stirrups for a Pap smear.

Also, your healthcare practitioner might not mind if you bring them with you. I never mind asking a nurse to take kids in the hall or behind the curtain during an exam. If you're not sure, call before your appointment and ask.

Patient: My boss won't let me off work.

My tough-love rebuttal: I understand that most people can't just up and quit their job when their boss is being unreasonable, but you really need to find a way to get to your appointment. Try to schedule the appointment months in advance so your boss can prepare for your absence. Ask if you can come in early or stay late to make up for the time. Or find a clinic that has early-morning, evening, or Saturday hours.

And, by the way, my sympathies for having the kind of boss who won't willingly give you time off to make sure you don't have cancer.

Patient: I get embarrassed during gynecology exams.

My tough-love rebuttal: I'm being sincere when I say this. As gynecologists, we examine thousands and thousands of patients during our career. It's true that no two are exactly the same, but if you've seen one vulva and vagina, you've pretty much seen them all. Please don't be embarrassed about any other part of the exam either. And there is no need to shave or shower before your appointment. Just come as you are. We just want to help you protect your health.

Patient: I don't really like going to the gynecologist.

My tough-love rebuttal: Sounds logical. If you did, I'd suggest that you reevaluate your entire life. Gynecology appointments aren't designed to be fun. We are not trying to entertain you. We're trying to keep you healthy. But, on another note, if you don't like going because of a past experience, please just let us know at the beginning of the appointment. Before the exam starts, you can even say, "If I say stop, do you promise you'll stop?" If your doctor can't make that promise, find a new one. You have a right to be in charge of what happens at all times.

I could include tons of other scenarios, but no matter what your excuse is, please trust and believe that I'd have a tough-love rebuttal that leads to the same conclusion: get your routine check-ups. So now that we've gotten that out of the way, let's talk about what you need to know to protect your breasts and your cervix.

CANCER PREVENTION CRASH COURSE
What You Need to Know to Patient Like a Pro

Breast Cancer Screening

Question 1: If I don't have a family history of breast cancer, do I still need to watch out for it?

Question 2: Should I be doing monthly breast self-exams?

Question 3: What should I know about breast cancer symptoms?

Question 4: What are some of the things that increase my risk of breast cancer?

Question 5: How often should I be screened?

Question 6: Are there any risks involved with getting a mammogram?

Cervical Cancer Screening

Question 7: What does a Pap smear check for?

Question 8: How often do I need to get Pap smears?

Question 9: Can I get a Pap or HPV test if I'm on my period?

Question 10: In the past, people got Pap smears when they became sexually active. Now they don't start until they're twenty-one. Plus, you're saying get them every three to five years instead of every year. Why do the Pap smear guidelines keep changing?

Breast Cancer Screening: What You Need to Know to Protect "Your Girls"

Question 1: If I don't have a family history of breast cancer, do I still need to watch out for it?

Yes. A lot of people know that approximately one in eight women in the United States will develop breast cancer in her lifetime. But what most people don't realize is that if I line up 10 women with breast cancer, only 1.5 of those women will have a family history of the disease. That means that about 85 percent of breast cancers occur in women who don't have a family history of it.[1] These cancers are not due to genetic mutations that these women were born with; rather, these cancers happen because of genetic mutations that happen as a result of the aging process and life in general. So even though you definitely need to tell your doc about your family history to determine your overall risk, all women (whether or not they have a family history) need to know about breast cancer detection and prevention.

Question 2: Should I be doing monthly breast self-exams?

This is going to surprise a lot of you, but over the years there has been some debate over how valuable monthly breast self-exams (BSEs) are for women who don't have a higher-than-normal risk of breast cancer. Basically, research came out saying that the masses that average-risk women find during BSEs lead to a higher rate of benign breast biopsies (and the anxiety that goes along with that process) but no decrease in breast cancer mortality rate. So a lot of important organizations, including the American Cancer Society, the US Preventive Services Task Force, and the American College of Obstetricians and Gynecologists, now advise against breast self-exams for women who don't have an increased risk of breast cancer.[2] Instead, they recommend something called breast self-awareness.

What's the difference between the two? With breast self-exams, you look for breast cancer by inspecting your breasts on a regular, repetitive basis. With breast self-awareness, there's not a strict guideline on the technique you should use or how frequently you should check your breasts. Instead, you focus on an overall awareness of how your breasts normally look and feel so you can easily notice if something changes.

So far no studies in the United States have looked at the effectiveness of breast self-awareness, but I can't wait to see those studies when they do come out. In the meantime, since approximately 50 percent of breast cancers in women fifty and older and 71 percent of breast cancers in women younger than fifty are detected by women themselves, I definitely don't recommend ignoring your breasts at home.[3] Know what's normal for you, and if you happen to notice any of the symptoms mentioned in the next question, or anything else that is concerning to you, definitely let your healthcare practitioner know. But remember that the breast self-awareness recommendation is for women with an *average* risk of breast cancer. If you have a higher-than-average risk of breast cancer (see question 5 for examples of high-risk individuals), continue breast self-exams unless your clinician tells you to stop them.

Question 3: What should I know about breast cancer symptoms?

There are three important things that I want you to remember. First of all, many breast cancers have no symptoms. None! Zero. Zilch. Nada. So even if you don't notice anything, you should still see your women's health practitioner regularly. Second, definitely tell your practitioner if you notice a breast mass, but don't panic. Most breast lumps are not breast cancer. And last but not least, not all breast cancers show up as lumps. Here are some other breast changes you might notice with breast cancer:[4]

- Thick areas of skin
- Skin dimpling
- Nipple crust
- Skin that is red, purplish, or warm to the touch
- Skin sores or irritation
- Nipple discharge other than breastmilk
- Growing vein
- Sunken nipple
- Change in breast size or shape
- Skin that looks like an orange peel
- Breast pain

Question 4: What are some of the things that increase my risk of breast cancer?

When it comes to preventing breast cancer, some risk factors are out of your control (such as being female, getting older, and having dense breasts). Here are some other factors to be aware of:

- **Drinking alcohol or smoking.** It's OK to drink occasionally; just don't make it a routine, because the more alcohol you drink, the higher your risk. Women who drink one alcoholic drink a day increase their breast cancer risk by 7 to 10 percent compared to non-drinkers. Women who have two to three drinks a day have about a 20 percent higher risk than nondrinkers. And pouring yourself "one big glass" isn't a way around that rule. One drink is defined as 5 ounces of wine, 1.5 ounces of liquor, or 12 ounces of beer. Smoking tobacco also increases your risk of breast cancer.
- **Being overweight or obese after menopause.** The link between weight and breast cancer risk is complex. The American Cancer Society recommends staying a healthy weight throughout life.
- **Being inactive.** Physical activity appears to reduce breast cancer risk, especially after menopause. Some studies show that even a little exercise every week may be helpful, but more seems better. The American Cancer Society suggests that adults get 75 minutes to 150 minutes of vigorous intensity or 150 to 300 minutes of moderate intensity activity each week (or a combination of these). If you are able to get more than 300 minutes of weekly exercise, that's ideal.
- **Not having children.** Women who do not have children or who have their first child after age thirty have a higher breast cancer risk.
- **Not breastfeeding.** Most research shows that breastfeeding decreases breast cancer risks, especially if it's done for a year or more.

- **Using some forms of birth control.** Estrogen-containing birth control pills may increase your breast cancer risk slightly. However, once the pills are stopped, the risk goes back to normal within about five to ten years. We don't have as many studies looking at the risk of breast cancer with skin patches and vaginal rings, but since they also contain estrogen and progestin, it is likely that they have the same effect on cancer risk. We don't have enough research to definitively say how progestin-only birth control impacts breast cancer risk; these options include progestin-only birth control pills, the birth control shot, the birth control implant, or progestin-containing IUDs.
- **Using hormone therapy.** There are two main types of hormone therapy (HT):
    - Estrogen plus progesterone, known as *combined hormone therapy*. If a woman still has a uterus, she needs progesterone in addition to estrogen (combined hormone therapy). This is because taking estrogen alone will increase her risk of uterine (endometrial) cancer. Using combined hormone therapy after menopause slightly increases the risk of breast cancer. The increased risk is usually seen after using it for approximately four years. When a woman uses this form of HT, there's also a higher likelihood that the cancer will be diagnosed at a more advanced stage. A woman's breast cancer risk seems to go back down within about five years of stopping this HT, but the increased risk does not completely go away.
    - Estrogen only. This is known as *estrogen therapy* (ET). This option is selected if a woman doesn't need endometrial protection because she has had

a hysterectomy. Some studies have found a slightly higher breast cancer risk, while others have found no increase in risk, or even a slight decrease in risk. If ET does increase the risk of breast cancer, it is not by a lot.

Question 5: How often should I be screened?

Based on their own interpretations of the risks versus benefits of earlier screening, different organizations have varying opinions when it comes to when you should start breast cancer screening and how often you should have it done. The chart below does not include all the reputable organizations who have recommendations, but I just want you to get a feel for how different they are.

Note: These recommendations are for women who are at *average risk*. If you are at an increased risk for any reason — for example, you have symptoms of breast cancer, a history of abnormal breast cells, certain genetic mutations like BRCA, a family history that puts you at a higher risk, or a personal history of chest radiation before the age of thirty — these recommendations don't apply to you. Your doctor will let you know how and when you should be screened.

Table 8. Breast Cancer Screening
Recommendations for Average-Risk Women[5]

	US Preventive Services Task Force	American Cancer Society	
Clinical breast exam (this is when a healthcare practitioner does the breast exam for you at your appointment instead of you doing it at home)	Insufficient evidence to recommend for or against	Does not recommend	
Mammography initiation age	Ages 40 to 49: initiate if the patient desires after being counseled; recommend at age 50	Ages 40 to 44: initiate if the patient desires after being counseled; recommend at age 45	
Mammography screening interval	Every two years	Ages 40 to 54: annual; ages 55 and older: every two years, or annual if desired by the patient	
Mammography stop age	The current evidence is insufficient to assess the balance of benefits and harms of screening mammograms in women 75 years and older	When life expectancy is less than 10 years	

	American College of Obstetricians and Gynecologists	National Comprehensive Cancer Network
	25 to 39 years old: may offer every 1 to 3 years; 40 years and older: may offer annually	25 to 39 years old: recommend every 1 to 3 years; 40 years and older: recommend annually
	Ages 40 to 49: initiate if the patient desires after being counseled; recommend at age 50	Age 40: recommend
	Annual or every two years	Annual
	After age 75, the decision to continue mammograms is based on a shared decision-making process that includes a discussion of the woman's health status and her longevity	When severe comorbidities limit life expectancy to 10 years or less

Question 6: Are there any risks involved with getting a mammogram?

Yes. But before we get to those, let me be very clear: mammograms save lives. When breast cancer is detected early, when it's small and hasn't spread, it's easier to treat it successfully. Getting screening tests regularly is the most reliable way to detect breast cancer early. I support mammograms 100 percent. With that said, here are the risks:

- **False positives.** Increased screening frequencies increase the probability of false-positive results (saying you have an abnormality when you don't). Those inaccurate results lead to repeat imaging or biopsies, and that causes anxiety and distress that doesn't always resolve, even if the follow-up testing is negative. The patient might also have to pay out of pocket for the additional workup.

- **Overdiagnosis and overtreatment.** In some cases, a cancer can remain indolent — meaning it will not progress to symptomatic cancer. Overdiagnosis happens when screening detects cancer that would not have progressed to symptomatic cancer.[6] Since it would be unethical to do a study that denied women treatment after they were diagnosed with breast cancer, we don't know exactly how frequently patients are overdiagnosed. But *do not* make a treatment decision based on the assumption that your cancer won't progress.

- **Radiation exposure.** According to a recent study, if you screen 100,000 women aged forty to seventy-four annually, the screening will cause 125 cases of breast cancer and sixteen cases of breast cancer death. But it will prevent 968 cancer deaths. So the benefits outweigh the risks by a lot.

- **Discomfort.** Mammograms are uncomfortable. Your breasts are compressed to flatten out the tissue. This decreases the amount of radiation needed to create the image and makes the image clearer.

There are two main types of mammograms currently available: 2D and 3D. During a 2D screening mammogram, two X-ray images are taken, one from the top and a second from the side. In a 3D screening mammogram, more images are taken. From a patient perspective, getting a 2D mammogram is very similar to getting a 3D mammogram: both require compression of the breast. However, since 3D mammograms provide more-detailed images, they decrease your chance of getting a false positive. In addition, they modestly increase the detection of breast cancer. Many insurance companies cover the cost of 3D mammograms.

DR. NITA'S NOTE
Ovarian Cancer and Endometrial Cancer Spotlight
Ovarian Cancer Screening

Who gets ovarian cancer? Half of all ovarian cancers are found in women who are sixty-three and older. Ovarian cancer is rare in women younger than forty.[7]

How common is it? In the United States, about twenty thousand women are diagnosed with ovarian cancer each year.

How can I get screened for it? If you are at high risk for ovarian cancer due to a strong family history or certain genetic mutations (like a BReast CAncer [BRCA] gene mutation or Lynch Syndrome), your doctor might recommend that you periodically have a transvaginal ultrasound to look for changes in your ovaries, and they might periodically draw your blood to check for a tumor marker called CA 125. However, these screening tests have a limited ability to find ovarian cancer at an early, more treatable stage. In addition to ultrasounds and CA 125 levels, in some cases, your doctor might also recommend surgical removal of your ovaries and fallopian tubes at a certain age or after you are finished with childbearing.

If you are a woman with an average risk of ovarian cancer and you don't have any symptoms, no screening strategy does a good job when it comes to detecting early-stage ovarian cancer.

As an average-risk woman who doesn't get screened, what should I look out for? The best way for you to protect yourself is to contact a healthcare professional if you have any of the following symptoms, especially if you have them for more than twelve days a month:

- Bloating or an increase in abdominal size
- Pelvic or abdominal pain
- Difficulty eating or feeling full quickly
- Urinary symptoms such as frequency (peeing a lot) and urgency
- Other symptoms include, but are not limited to, menstrual changes, postmenopausal bleeding, or abnormal vaginal discharge

Of course, having these symptoms doesn't automatically mean that you have ovarian cancer, but it's a good idea to find out what's causing them. For instance, urinary tract infections are a much more common cause of urinary frequency and urgency. And bloating can be caused by gastrointestinal issues.

Endometrial Cancer Screening

Who gets endometrial cancer? Endometrial cancer (cancer of the inside lining of the uterus) can happen to women of younger ages, but most cases are diagnosed in women who are past menopause and are in their mid-sixties. This cancer is more common in Black women than white women, and Black women are more likely to die from it.

How common is it? Endometrial cancer is the most common type of cancer that affects the female reproductive organs. In the United States, approximately sixty thousand new cases of endometrial cancer are diagnosed each year.

How can I get screened for it? If you are at high risk for endometrial cancer because of a genetic mutation like Lynch syndrome, your doctor might periodically biopsy the inside lining of your uterus. In some cases, a hysterectomy (removal of the uterus) is recommended after you have completed childbearing.[8]

But if you are a woman with an average risk, there is no effective screening for endometrial cancer.

As an average-risk woman who doesn't get screened, what should I look out for? The most common sign of endometrial cancer is abnormal bleeding. If you are postmenopausal, any vaginal bleeding should be evaluated to rule out cancer. If you are premenopausal, your doctor will determine if you need to be evaluated for cancer. Regardless of age, being overweight or obese increases a person's chance of getting endometrial cancer.

Cervical Cancer Screening: No More Yearly Paps

Question 7: What does a Pap smear check for?

During a papanicolaou (pa-puh-NEE-kel-ow) smear — better known as a Pap smear, Pap test, or cervical cytology — a practitioner inserts a speculum to give a clear view of the cervix (see figure 13). Cells are removed from the cervix with a brush or other sampling instrument, and the cells are sent to the laboratory to check for cervical cancer, precancer, and/or high-risk human papillomavirus (HPV).

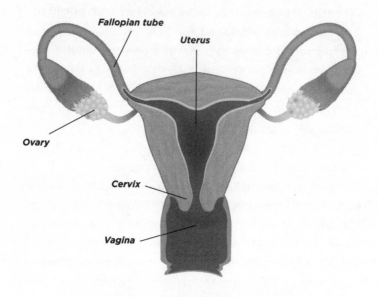

Figure 13. Female anatomy

Some patients incorrectly believe that a Pap smear will also screen them for ovarian cancer or endometrial cancer (cancer of the inside lining of the uterus). Yes, it's true that on rare occasions, ovarian cancer cells travel away from the ovaries, through the fallopian tubes and uterus, and then down to the cervix, where they *happen* to be detected on a Pap smear. And it's also true that sometimes abnormal endometrial cells *happen* to be detected on a Pap. But a Pap's claim to fame is cervical cancer screening. It is *not* a reliable screening test for ovarian or endometrial cancer.

Question 8: How often do I need to get Pap smears?

The following women may not need regular Pap or HPV tests:

- Women older than sixty-five who have had negative screenings during the past ten years, with the most recent test happening within the past five years, and who have been told by their doctors that they don't need to be tested anymore
- Women who do not have a cervix (usually because of a hysterectomy) and have no history of cervical cancer or abnormal Pap test results

Always talk to your healthcare practitioner before stopping Pap and HPV tests.

And for everyone else...

Even if you received all your HPV vaccine shots, you've never been sexually active, or you've gone through menopause, these guidelines still apply to you:

- Women ages twenty-one to twenty-nine get a Pap every three years.
- Women thirty to sixty-five get:
  - a Pap test every three years, *or*
  - a high-risk HPV test every five years (an HPV test looks for DNA from HPV in cells from your cervix), *or*
  - a Pap test and a high-risk HPV test together (co-testing) every five years.
- High-risk HPV testing can be considered for women who are twenty-five to twenty-nine, but Pap tests are preferred.

If your cervical cancer screening is abnormal, you may need to have Pap tests more frequently than what's listed above. Your doctor may also recommend a test called colposcopy, which is when we look at the abnormal areas on your cervix with a light and a magnifier (called a colposcope). During colposcopy, your practitioner may perform a biopsy (remove a sample of tissue from your cervix) to check for precancerous or cancerous cells. The results of the biopsy will help determine the best treatment option(s) for you.

Your doctor or nurse may also recommend more frequent testing if you have a weakened immune system because of an organ transplant, chemotherapy, or steroid use; if you are living with HIV/AIDS; or if your mother or grandmother took a medication called diethylstilbestrol (DES) while pregnant. (DES was prescribed to pregnant women in the United States between 1940 and 1971 to prevent miscarriage, premature labor, and other complications of pregnancy. Daughters, and possibly granddaughters, of women who took DES while pregnant with them have a higher risk of cervical cancer as well as some other types of cancer.)

Note: If a person between the ages of twenty-one and twenty-nine has an abnormal Pap smear, sometimes we will check their high-risk HPV status. However, the reason we usually do Paps instead of HPV testing or cotesting for cervix owners between twenty-one and twenty-nine is that high-risk HPV is very common in this age group, but their immune systems usually clear the virus within one to two years (before the virus has a chance to cause cancer). Therefore, we don't need to subject them to medical procedures for HPV infections that will resolve without causing long-term harmful changes in cervical cells. In women aged thirty to sixty-five, the presence of HPV at the cervix is more likely to turn into cancer. So checking for HPV in that age group is important.

Question 9: Can I get a Pap or HPV test if I'm on my period?

Yes. However, ideally, you should schedule your appointment when you do not expect to have your period. This is because if your flow is heavy, your period might affect the results of the Pap or HPV test. But it's better to get a Pap while you're on your period than to not get one at all. If you are not sure or if you feel uncomfortable, call your nurse or doctor before your appointment.

Question 10: In the past, people got Pap smears when they became sexually active. Now they don't start until they're twenty-one. Plus, you're saying get them every three to five years instead of every year. Why do the Pap smear guidelines keep changing?

As new research comes out, the guidelines change periodically. I know it can get confusing. I tell patients to keep coming, and we'll keep them up to date on what the latest research recommends.

DR. NITA'S NOTE

Advocate for Your Health Like a Pro for Breast and Cervical Cancer Prevention

Breast Care

1. Make sure your doctor knows about any family history of cancer, no matter what kind it is. You may only think to tell your doctor about female cancers, but sometimes other parts of your family history can provide valuable clues.
2. Tell your doctor about any known genetic mutations in your family. Remember that genetic conditions can be passed down from your mom or dad.
3. Ask if anything in your personal or family history makes

you need imaging for breast cancer screening earlier or more frequently than what's recommended for women with an average risk for cancer. See question 5 (page 257) for a summary of the current recommendations.

4. If you are thirty-five or older, ask your doctor about the Gail model at your next wellness appointment. This is a free online tool that quickly estimates your risk of developing invasive breast cancer over the next five years and up to age ninety. However, know that there are a number of limitations to the Gail model. Although a woman's risk may be accurately estimated, the predictions do not precisely predict which woman will develop breast cancer. In fact, some women who do not develop breast cancer have higher risk estimates than some women who do eventually develop breast cancer. Also, the Gail model cannot estimate breast cancer risks in women who have a BRCA1 or BRCA2 mutation or a history of invasive breast cancer, or who are in certain other groups. If you can't use the Gail model, your clinician may be able to suggest a different model that can estimate your breast cancer risk.

5. Do away with the "no news is good news" mentality. Make sure you see a written report confirming that your mammogram was normal. If you have an abnormal result, print it out or ask for a copy of it so you can always have easy access to that information if you switch doctors in the future. And if you have any breast biopsies, make sure you keep a copy of the pathology report(s).

6. If you have an abnormal mammogram, always follow up as instructed.

Pro tip: Currently, doctors still frequently rely on CDs to view images that were taken at outside facilities. Therefore, when you arrive for your mammogram appointment, always request a CD with your mammogram images on it. If you go to another facility in the future, you can let them copy the CD. Having previous mammograms to compare your imaging to will decrease the chance of you getting called back for repeat imaging. They usually give you the CD immediately after your mammogram is completed. (Note: This CD, which is usually free, is not the same as the written report that tells you whether your mammogram was normal. You should get the written report a week or two after your mammogram.)

Pap Tests

1. Ask if you are getting a Pap test, HPV testing, or co-testing. See question 8 (page 265) if you need a refresher on these terms.
2. If you want STD screening, let your practitioner know. They can easily test for gonorrhea, chlamydia, or trichomoniasis during your Pap smear.
3. At the end of your appointment, ask when you should have another Pap test (assuming your results are normal that day). But if your Pap test that is being done that day comes back abnormal, you will need to follow up sooner.
4. Ask for a copy of your Pap test result. As with mammograms, do away with the "no news is good news" mentality. If you have an abnormal result, print it out or ask for a copy of it so you can always have easy access to that information if you switch doctors in the future. And if you need follow-up procedures/biopsies because of an abnormal Pap, keep those records/pathology reports too.
5. If you have an abnormal Pap, always follow up as instructed.

Extra #DrNitaNotes to help you put all the information together

Ultimately, I want you to be informed enough to make the right decision for yourself, but (just in case you're wondering) based on all the info and research I've seen, this is what I currently recommend for women who have a cervix and are not at an increased risk for breast or cervical cancer:

Ages 21 to 24

- Breast self-awareness
- Pap test every 3 years

Ages 25 to 29

- Breast self-awareness
- Clinical breast exam every 1 to 3 years
- Pap test every 3 years

Ages 30 to 39

- Breast self-awareness
- Clinical breast exam every 1 to 3 years
- Pap and high-risk HPV test every 5 years *or* high-risk HPV test every 5 years

Ages 40 to 49

- Breast self-awareness
- Mammogram and clinical breast exam every year
- Pap test and high-risk HPV test every 5 years *or* high-risk HPV test every 5 years

Ages 50 and older

- Breast self-awareness
- Mammogram and clinical breast exam every year until you are 75 *or* your life expectancy is less than 10 years
- Pap test and high-risk HPV test every 5 years *or* high-risk HPV test every 5 years. Talk to your doctor about whether you need to be screened after 65.

Chapter 12

Pee and Stuff

Urinary Incontinence

"It's possible that your date had a micropenis. That's a rare condition where an adult male's stretched penis is 3.67 inches or less."

I was at dinner with four friends, and that was my response to one of the many burning questions they had during our girl's night out — which had somehow turned into an "Ask Dr. Nita" seminar. Everybody at the table was emotionally invested as they asked question after question and listened to my detailed medical explanations about bumping, grinding, and being dickmatized — which is when the penis is so good that you start to catch feelings for a guy. But after I mentioned that a lot of women struggle with urinary incontinence, my same friends who had a million and one questions about how to fix different sexual problems just kinda shrugged and said something along the lines of, "It happens to me all the time, but what are you gonna do? That's just life."

But actually, contrary to popular belief, it doesn't have to be this way! It's true that your risk of incontinence increases as you get older, but incontinence is not a normal part of aging.

We have some fantastic medical treatments that can improve (and sometimes totally resolve) urinary incontinence. As a woman, you don't have to walk around peeing on yourself.

So if you're longing for a life that doesn't involve daily panty liners, incontinence pads, or adult diapers, this chapter is for you.

URINARY ISSUES CRASH COURSE
What You Need to Know to Patient Like a Pro

Question 1: I'm grown. I really don't want to tell my doctor I'm peeing on myself. Why shouldn't I be embarrassed?

Question 2: You said urinary incontinence is common. How common?

Question 3: Am I leaking urine because of a dangerous underlying issue?

Question 4: I haven't noticed any of the things mentioned in question number 3 with my urinary incontinence. What's the most likely cause for me?

Question 5: How can my healthcare practitioner figure out which type of incontinence I have?

Question 6: What are some medicine-free and surgery-free options that might help if my doctor tells me that I have stress, urge, or mixed incontinence?

Question 7: Dr. Nita, I tried medicine-free and surgery-free recommendations for six weeks to six months, but I'm still having stress incontinence. What's next for me?

Question 8: What do you recommend if I tried medicine-free and surgery-free recommendations for six weeks to six months, but I still have urge incontinence or overactive bladder symptoms?

Question 9: I have mixed incontinence. What should I consider after conservative treatment options fail?

Question 10: I've been treated for UTIs repeatedly, but I keep having symptoms. Why is that happening?

Question 1: I'm grown. I really don't want to tell my doctor I'm peeing on myself. Why shouldn't I be embarrassed?

Urinary incontinence, also known as accidental bladder leak-age, is so common that a lot of gynecologists are required to spend months (literally … months) of their training learning about incontinence issues and how to treat them. Then, after finishing a four-year ob-gyn training program, some doctors decide to learn even more about the subject by going into a subspecialty called urogynecology — *uro* means relating to urine or the urinary organs. That means these doctors enjoy helping people with urinary issues so much that they become a "urine gynecologist." Well, *urogynecologist* (not urine gynecologist) is the official term, but you get my point. In addition, doctors called urologists also specialize in urinary issues, and internal medicine/family practice doctors see a lot of urinary incontinence patients too.

There's nothing to be embarrassed about. Incontinence is very common.

Question 2: You said urinary incontinence is common. How common?

We see incontinence all. the. time. Estimates vary, but some research shows that up to 70 percent of women have incontinence at some point in their life. And it can start at a young age. In one study, more than 25 percent of young female athletes participating in high-impact sports reported experiencing incontinence, but more than 90 percent of them had never told anyone about their problem and had no knowledge about how they could prevent it from happening.[1]

Question 3: Am I leaking urine because of a dangerous underlying issue?

If your leaking starts suddenly or if any of the following happens with your urinary incontinence, a doctor should make sure that you don't have a serious underlying medical issue:

- Numbness
- Leg weakness
- Stool leakage
- Seeing blood in your urine
- Multiple UTIs (three or more in a year)
- Pain
- Fever
- Difficulty urinating or emptying your bladder when you actually try to
- Incontinence that happens without a preceding urge to urinate

Pro tip: If you are referred to a specialist for further evaluation, bring all your records pertaining to your urinary issue with you in paper or electronic form, including urine culture results.

Question 4: I haven't noticed any of the things mentioned in question number 3 with my urinary incontinence. What's the most likely cause for me?

Since this is a crash course, I'll focus on the main three reasons that women experience urinary incontinence:

- **Stress incontinence.** This type of incontinence happens when the muscles and tissue around the urethra (the tube where urine exits) are not strong enough to stay closed when there is increased pressure ("stress") in the abdomen (see figure 14). Women with stress incontinence have leakage during activities like coughing, laughing, sneezing, running, lifting things, bending over, having sex, or even just walking. When people say, "Don't make me laugh, I'm gonna pee myself," this is the type of incontinence they are usually experiencing.

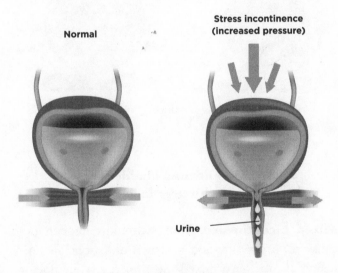

Normal

Stress incontinence (increased pressure)

Urine

Figure 14. A normal bladder versus a bladder with stress urinary incontinence

- **Urge incontinence.** With this type of incontinence, your sudden urge to urinate is so strong that you can't hold your urine long enough to get to the toilet. Most people experience urge incontinence because their bladder muscles randomly squeeze before their bladder is full (see figure 15). People with urge incontinence may experience leakage when they unlock their front door when returning home or when they hear water running.

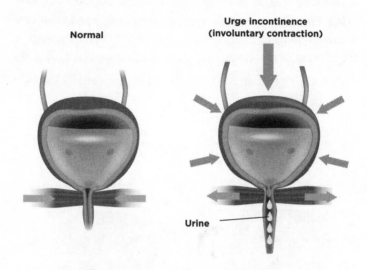

Normal

Urge incontinence (involuntary contraction)

Urine

Figure 15. A normal bladder versus a bladder with urge incontinence

- **Mixed incontinence.** Your symptoms happen because of a combination of stress and urge incontinence. If you have mixed incontinence, your doctor will probably start off by focusing on the type of incontinence that bothers you the most.

With urinary incontinence, some people just release a few drops; others end up with completely soaked underwear.

DR. NITA'S NOTE
Overactive Bladder Syndrome

As stated above, people with *urge urinary incontinence* have a sudden urge to pee right before they accidentally leak urine. People with *overactive bladder (OAB) syndrome* feel a sudden urge to pee; *plus*, many of them need to urinate a lot during the day and night. They may or may not have urge urinary incontinence.

There are two kinds of overactive bladder: The type that doesn't involve urge incontinence is called *overactive bladder, dry*. The type that does involve urge incontinence is called *overactive bladder, wet*. Therefore, a person may or may not have urinary incontinence with OAB.

Like people with urge incontinence, people with OAB may notice an urge to urinate when they unlock their front door when returning home or when they hear water running. OAB is typically treated the same way as urge incontinence.

The terms *urge incontinence* and *overactive bladder with incontinence* are often used interchangeably.

Question 5: How can my healthcare practitioner figure out which type of incontinence I have?

First of all, ask your doctor to look at your list of medications. For example, the following may be causing or contributing to your incontinence.

- antihistamines like Benadryl
- muscle relaxants and sedatives

- narcotics
- diuretics (water pills)

Your doctor should also make sure that a medical condition, such as a UTI or diabetes, isn't to blame. If those issues aren't the culprit, it's helpful if you have a bladder diary to review. A bladder diary, also known as a voiding diary, is a simple chart that allows you to write down the following:

- Amount of fluid you drink (you will need a jug with milliliter [mL] increments)
- How much urine you make (you will need a second jug that's at least 500 mL to measure your urine; this jug should also be in mL increments)
- Any accidental urine leakage, along with what you were doing when the leaking happened

You collect the information for twenty-four hours at a time. The bladder diary should be completed over three days, but those days don't have to be consecutive. The next page has an example of a shortened version of a bladder diary. If you'd like to complete a bladder diary, do an internet search for "free bladder diary template."

Date:

Time	Drinks		Urine		Leakage		
	Amount (mL)	Type	Amount (mL)	How urgent, on a scale from 0 to 3 (3 = extremely urgent)	Leakage with urgency	Leakage with activities	Amount, 1 to 3 (3 = fully soaked pad)
7:00 a.m.			200 mL	0			
8:00 a.m.	250 mL	Coffee					
9:00 a.m.			100 mL	3	Y		2
10:00 a.m.	500 mL	Water					
11:00 a.m.						cough	2

Your doctor might be able to determine your diagnosis after looking at your bladder diary and listening to your history. Or sometimes they will do a physical exam and/or something called a cough stress test, which is when you are asked to cough with a full bladder while your healthcare practitioner watches for urine leakage. In some cases, if the diagnosis is not clear or they are planning surgery they might also recommend additional testing such as urodynamics, which is an in-office test that looks at how well your bladder, sphincters, and urethra work to store and release urine. If you need urodynamics, it will probably be done by a gynecologist, urogynecologist, or a urologist. During urodynamics, small catheters are placed inside your bladder and rectum to determine how much urine your bladder can hold, what causes you to leak urine, and how your bladder empties. The small catheters used during urodynamics might cause a little discomfort, but it's not a painful procedure.

DR. NITA'S NOTE
Urinary Tract Infection (UTI) Spotlight

What is a UTI? An infection in any part of the urinary tract — the urethra (the tube where pee exits), bladder, ureters (tubes that carry urine from the kidneys to the bladder), or kidneys.

What causes a UTI? It usually happens because bacteria have made it into your urethra. Then, if urination doesn't flush out the bacteria or your immune system can't fight the bacteria off before they have a chance to take hold and grow, you officially have a UTI.

What are some possible symptoms? Below are the most common ones, but note that some people don't have any UTI symptoms.

- Dysuria, or pain while peeing. But if you notice a change in your vaginal discharge or vaginal itching in addition to the dysuria, a UTI might not be to blame. A vaginal infection (like yeast or a sexually transmitted disease) may be causing your symptoms.
- Frequency — you have to pee all the time, even when you have only a little urine to pass.
- Urgency — when you have to pee, you have to go urgently.
- Uncomfortable pelvic pressure or pelvic/back cramping.
- Blood in your urine (red, pink, or cola-colored).
- Pee that smells like a kitty litter box (or ammonia) or looks cloudy.
- Urinary incontinence.

How is a UTI usually treated if it's contained to the bladder? Your doctor will give you a one- to seven-day course of antibiotics. (Note: Don't think your doctor is "shortchanging" you if you get one of the shorter courses of antibiotics. Some antibiotics are known to get the job done more quickly.)

What if you get recurrent UTIs after sex? Try the following. (You can use these tips even if your UTIs are not specifically linked to sex.)

1. **Behavior/lifestyle changes.** If you're looking for pill-free suggestions, give these a try.
   - Drink more water. Drink two liters of water a day to flush out your urinary tract.
   - Use something besides spermicides for birth control.

   We don't have solid research to back these next two recommendations, but you can give them a try:

   - Empty your bladder right before and right after sex.

(If this doesn't seem to help after a few months, feel free to stop interrupting your post-sex cuddle time.)

o   Wipe from front to back.

2. **Vaginal estrogen.** If you fall into one of the following categories, ask your healthcare practitioner if vaginal estrogen might be helpful for you:

o   You are menopausal or you are getting close to menopause.

o   You are postpartum and/or breastfeeding.

o   You are using hormonal birth control.

All of those situations can lower your estrogen level, which can result in more UTIs. Of note, vaginal estrogen is not the same as systemic estrogen; vaginal estrogen stays local.

3. **Additional strategies.**

o   Cranberry products (including juice, capsules, and tablets). Cranberry products don't cure UTIs, but they might help prevent UTIs by stopping bacteria from adhering to the bladder wall. For cranberry products to be effective, you need at least 36 mg of proanthocyanidins (PACs). So if you buy a supplement, make sure that the label says "36 mg PACs per dose." If you opt for cranberry juice, get the sourest kind you can find. But be aware that even sour cranberry juice has a lot of sugar, and sugar can make your symptoms worse.

o   Methenamine salts with vitamin C. Methenamine is an antibacterial medicine. The recommended dosing for this option is typically 1 g of methenamine hippurate orally twice daily. Additionally, you take 1 to 2 g of vitamin C for every 1 g of methenamine salt.

o   Probiotics. If you choose to use a probiotic, consider Lactobacillus rhamnosus or Lactobacillus reuteri.

- ○ D-mannose. This option tends to work best if your recurrent UTIs are caused by a bacteria called E. coli.

  If you want to give supplements a try, remember that the FDA does not require supplement makers to prove that their products are safe and/or effective before selling them.

4. **Take an antibiotic after sex.** If you repeatedly develop bladder infections (i.e., two or more UTIs within six months) and you aren't able to stop them with the preventive tips above, you may benefit from postcoital prophylaxis, which is when you take a single dose of an antibiotic within two hours after sex to keep a UTI from coming on. If a patient chooses this option, I ask them to come back after about three months of treatment to make sure they're happy with the regimen. Many women keep using the antibiotic for months or years, but there are potential risks associated with long-term antibiotic use, including but not limited to vaginal and oral yeast infections, antibiotic drug resistance, and reducing the number of good bacteria in your gut. You should understand the risks, benefits, and alternatives before starting long-term antibiotic treatment.

   The choice of antibiotic is based on how susceptible the bacteria from your previous infections have been to treatment, your history of drug allergies, and the potential for interactions with other medications you may be taking. (Note: For repeat UTIs not specifically related to sex, your doctor can still recommend prophylaxis options.)

Question 6: What are some medicine-free and surgery-free options that might help if my doctor tells me that I have stress, urge, or mixed incontinence?

You can try these recommendations for six weeks to six months.

- **Maintain an ideal body weight.** If you are overweight or obese, talk to your healthcare practitioner about weight loss strategies: since excess weight puts extra pressure on the bladder and pelvic muscles. Losing weight can help or even eliminate stress incontinence. It can also help to improve chronic medical conditions that increase the likelihood of incontinence (like high blood pressure or diabetes). Studies show that more than 80 percent of obese or overweight women notice incontinence improvement with weight loss!

- **Do Kegels (correctly).** If your doctor confirms that you have weak pelvic-floor muscles, Kegels can be very helpful. However, most women clench their abs, buttocks, or thigh muscles instead of their pelvic muscles when they are attempting to do Kegels. Doing Kegels wrong and expecting your pelvic muscles to get stronger is like working on your biceps at the gym but expecting your triceps to bulk up. If you are having a hard time finding the right muscles, ask your doctor to make sure you're doing them correctly. By placing one or two fingers in your vagina and asking you to contract the pelvic-floor muscles that you typically use to stop urine or bowel gas, they are able to check your technique during a pelvic exam. In some instances, to help you improve your Kegel technique they might recommend weighted vaginal cones, pelvic physical therapy, and/or something called biofeedback, which places pressure sensors in the vagina to measure pressure to let you know when you are using the correct muscles. There are also lots of apps and devices that can help you with your exercises. As a cohost on *The Doctors*, I tried out a vaginal device that allowed me to control video games with my pelvic floor. It was the most fun I've ever had while doing Kegels.

Kegels can strengthen your pelvic muscles to help with stress incontinence. But they also come in handy with urge incontinence. If you feel a sudden urge to urinate, using the "freeze-and-squeeze" technique can decrease bladder contractions and give you more time to get to the toilet. To do this, you freeze (stop what you are doing) and squeeze (do three Kegels).

Here are some brief instructions for how to do them correctly:

1. Squeeze your pelvic-floor muscles. To find the right muscles, pretend you are trying to hold in a fart on the elevator.
2. Keep contracting them for three to five seconds (or as long as you can).
3. Relax for three to five seconds.
4. Try to do three sets of eight to twelve Kegels a day. (Your healthcare practitioner can talk to you about your specific situation and whether you should follow a different regimen.)

- **Train your bladder.** With bladder training, you urinate on a schedule instead of waiting until your bladder is very full. Bladder training is most effective for women with urgency incontinence, but some women who have stress incontinence that only happens at higher bladder volumes may also benefit from the timed voiding to keep bladder volumes below the level where stress incontinence occurs. For details on how to go about bladder training, see appendix C.

- **Take it easy with liquids.** Most people don't need to consume more than 48 to 64 ounces of liquids a day from all sources (including beverages, soup, etc.). However, if you need to drink more for medical reasons or if you are sweating because you are active or it is hot, listen to your body. Don't restrict your fluids so much that you are walking around thirsty or dehydrated. Your pee will also clue you in. If you have dark, concentrated urine, you need to drink more water.
- **Treat your constipation.** Being constipated can make incontinence worse. So make sure you are drinking enough water and try to incorporate fiber-rich foods. Eating more whole-grain foods has turned some of my constipated patients into pooping powerhouses.
- **Change your diet.** Minimize bladder irritants like alcohol, caffeine, spicy foods, artificial sweeteners, and carbonated beverages.
- **Stop smoking.** Tobacco is a bladder irritant. Plus, coughing puts pressure on the bladder. Less smoking means less coughing.

Ideally, you want to find a treatment option that will eliminate the need for pads, but until you are accident-free I recommend wearing incontinence pads instead of menstrual pads because menstrual pads don't absorb urine well. If you are sensitive to pads, there are also underwear that absorb urine to eliminate wetness and smell. Whatever you use, change your incontinence product frequently because chronic exposure to urine can result in skin irritation and breakdown.

DR. NITA'S NOTE
Pelvic Organ Prolapse Spotlight

With pelvic organ prolapse (POP), your pelvic-floor muscles become too lax. And because of that, your bladder, rectum, intestines, or uterus/vaginal vault drop lower in the pelvis. So on a fundamental level, pelvic organ prolapse means that one or more of your pelvic organs is falling out — either a little bit or a lot.

Here are the technical terms we use to specify which organ is no longer in its rightful place (and see figure 16):

- *Cystocele*, pronounced SIS-tuh-seal. This is when your bladder bulges into or beyond your vaginal walls.
- *Rectocele*, pronounced REC-tuh-seal. This is when your rectum bulges into or beyond your vaginal walls.
- *Enterocele* (EN-ter-o-seal). This is when your intestines bulge into or beyond your vaginal walls.
- *Apical compartment prolapse.* This is when whatever is at the apex (top) of your vagina bulges into or beyond your vaginal walls. This could be either your uterus and cervix, your cervix alone, or your vaginal vault, depending on whether you've had a hysterectomy.

What are the symptoms? Many women with POP don't have any symptoms. Those who do may complain of vaginal or pelvic pressure and/or feeling like they have a vaginal bulge or something falling out of their vagina. Some may also feel aching in the pelvis or lower back. Symptoms usually worsen with standing and activity. Which makes sense because... gravity. Patients may also notice urinary incontinence, difficulty emptying their bladder when they actually want to, problems with constipation, or incomplete bowel emptying.

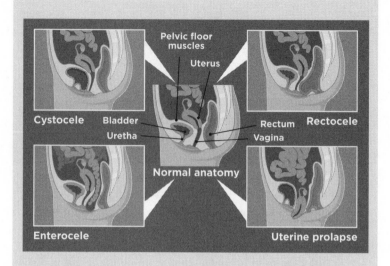

Figure 16. Types of pelvic organ prolapse

Why does it happen? Risk factors for pelvic organ prolapse include:[2]

- **Pregnancy.** The more pregnancies, the higher the chance of prolapse in the future. It's not clear whether having a C-section prevents prolapse.
- **Advancing age.** Most women who complain of pelvic organ prolapse are in their sixties or seventies. However, some women can experience it earlier.
- **Obesity.** Compared to normal-weight peers, overweight and obese women have a nearly 40 to 50 percent increased risk of pelvic organ prolapse.
- **Hysterectomy.** The role of hysterectomy in the development of subsequent POP is controversial. Factors like surgical technique may play a role.
- **Race and ethnicity.** Some, but not all, studies show that the risk of pelvic organ prolapse is lower in

African American women and higher in white and Latina women.

- **Other.** Chronic constipation, repetitive heavy lifting, and genetics.

What are the treatment options? Some people's prolapse is barely noticeable during exams, but sometimes a person's prolapsed organ can literally be seen hanging out of their vagina. The severity of your prolapse determines which treatment options will work for you. Here are some things that can help:

- **Kegels.** In mild cases, *correctly* doing Kegels at home might be all you need.
- **Pelvic physical therapy.** If your prolapse isn't too severe, working with a pelvic physical therapist who teaches you how to strengthen your pelvic muscles might do the trick.
- **Vaginal pessary.** An option for mild, moderate, or really severe prolapse is a vaginal pessary — a silicone device that fits into your vagina to push any bulging organs back into place. Since these come in different shapes and sizes, your doctor will do a pessary fitting before ordering yours to see what size corrects your prolapse and feels comfortable. Some pessaries can even help with urinary incontinence. Most of my patients who choose a pessary are in their sixties and beyond. Younger people tend to prefer surgery.
- **Surgery.** If you are not planning to have children in the future and your doctor thinks you are healthy enough to be a good surgical candidate, you could also choose to have surgery to put any bulging organs back where they belong and to strengthen the tissues that keep them in place. Some surgical procedures are

done through the vagina, and others are done through an abdominal incision.

Prolapse is annoying, but it won't kill you. So if your symptoms are not bothersome, and the prolapse isn't causing a major issue (like preventing you from being able to pee), not getting treated won't impact your health.

Question 7: Dr. Nita, I tried medicine-free and surgery-free recommendations for six weeks to six months, but I'm still having stress incontinence. What's next for me?

Continue the medicine-free and surgery-free recommendations, but ask your doctor if one or more of the following might be a good option for you:

- **Vaginal estrogen.** This treatment is frequently helpful for women with stress incontinence who are menopausal or in the menopause transition. If a woman needs it, vaginal estrogen is usually offered with the medicine-free recommendations in question 6. But if you're using estrogen for incontinence, make sure it's vaginal estrogen since systemic (oral) menopausal hormone therapy may worsen urinary incontinence.
- **Pelvic-floor physical therapy.** If you haven't seen a qualified pelvic-floor physical therapist yet, you might benefit from going to some sessions to make sure you are doing your Kegels correctly.

- **"Incontinence tampons."** These can be purchased over the counter. This device comes in a tampon-style applicator. But instead of being a wad of absorbent fibers, they are collapsible silicone structures that lift and support the urethra to help prevent stress incontinence leaks.

- **Vaginal pessary.** This is a flexible device that's placed in the vagina to help prevent urinary incontinence (older patients who are poor surgical candidates or who want to avoid surgery usually use this option). Pessaries need to be removed and cleaned periodically. Some women do this themselves every week or two at home, and others choose to come into the clinic every three to six months for a pessary cleaning. Some pessaries can be left in place during sex but others can't. If you want your pessary out when you have sex, your doctor can show you how to take it out and put it back in. There is a small risk of irritation or erosion of the vaginal mucosa with any type of pessary, and the risk is higher if it's not cleaned regularly. If you experience irritation or erosion, vaginal estrogen and more frequent cleaning may be recommended.

- **Medications.** Currently, no medications are FDA approved to specifically treat stress incontinence. However, a lot of meds have been evaluated. Ask your doctor if they know of a medication that might be appropriate for you.

- **Bulking agent injections.** If the cause of your incontinence is weak tissue around the urethra, during this procedure, which is sometimes done in the doctor's office, a urologist or urogynecologist numbs your urethra and then injects a filler material (bulking agent) into the tissue around the urethra to prevent you from leaking with activities. This is like lip fillers for your urethra. The upside is that you won't have any incisions and there's no downtime. The downside is that it's not as effective as traditional surgery for stress urinary incontinence.

- **Traditional surgery.** Of all the treatment options, this is going to be the one that gives you the highest likelihood of success. Many different surgical procedures can help stress incontinence. The most common procedure is something called a "midurethral sling." This is when a narrow piece of synthetic mesh is placed under the urethra. It acts as a hammock to lift or support the urethra to help prevent stress incontinence leaks.

Going into detail about all the available surgeries goes beyond the scope of this crash course, so make sure you inquire about all your surgical options. And ask about the risks, benefits, and risk of failure of any surgical option that is suggested to you.

Surgeries are usually not recommended for people who plan to get pregnant again in the future since pregnancy and childbirth can disrupt the surgical repair and that can cause you to start leaking again. Bulking injections are an excellent option for these individuals.

Other options

- **Vaginal laser treatment.** This procedure is typically performed in the office with topical anesthesia. While some experts recommend laser treatment, others feel that more well-designed studies are needed to prove that this is an effective treatment option. Studies are currently ongoing. This procedure is generally not covered by insurance and typically comes with a hefty price tag.

- **Intravesical balloon device.** *Vesical* refers to the bladder, and for this treatment, a small balloon device is inserted into the bladder. Basically, the balloon acts as a "shock absorber" to decrease the temporary pressure changes in the bladder that are causing incontinence. We have a limited amount of research on the effectiveness of this option.

Question 8: What do you recommend if I tried medicine-free and surgery-free recommendations for six weeks to six months, but I still have urge incontinence or overactive bladder symptoms?

Continue the medicine-free and surgery-free recommendations, but ask your doctor if one or more of these might be a good option for you:

- **Vaginal estrogen** is sometimes helpful for women with urge incontinence who are menopausal or in the menopause transition. If a woman needs it, vaginal estrogen is usually offered with the medicine-free recommendations in question 6. But if you're using estrogen for incontinence, make sure it's vaginal estrogen since systemic (oral) menopausal hormone therapy may worsen urinary incontinence.
- **Pelvic-floor physical therapy.** If you haven't seen a qualified pelvic-floor physical therapist yet, you might benefit from going to some sessions to ensure that you are doing your Kegels correctly.
- **An oral medication** can be added. For example, Beta-3-adrenergic agonist or antimuscarinic agents are frequently used. You may see improvement in one or two weeks, but it may take up to twelve weeks for you to

notice a full response to the med(s). If you aren't happy with the initial medication, your doctor can increase your dose, switch you to a different medication (e.g., give you an antimuscarinic agent instead of a beta-3 adrenergic agonist), or combine a beta3-adrenergic agonist with an antimuscarinic. Make sure you understand the potential side effects and risks of the medication you choose. Your insurance coverage or cost may limit your options.

If you don't like the side effects or risks of the drugs, or if you can't find a drug regimen that relieves your symptoms to your satisfaction, ask your doctor about one of the following options.

- **Botox injection in the bladder.** This procedure helps stop unwanted bladder muscle contractions. It can be done under local anesthesia in the office. Results start to show after about two weeks and may last between three and twelve months. (Insurance may cover this after other treatment options have been ineffective for you.)

- **Percutaneous tibial nerve stimulation.** During this in-office procedure, an acupuncture-like needle is placed behind the ankle and mild electrical stimulation is administered for thirty minutes. Sessions occur once a week for twelve weeks and then approximately once a month for maintenance (although the optimal maintenance schedule is not known). This works by impacting the nerves that supply the bladder. Alternatively, an implantable tibial nerve stimulation device with a three-to-five-year battery life called eCoin was also recently approved by the FDA. There is also an at-home option for this, called transcutaneous tibial nerve stimulation (TTNS). TTNS uses a noninvasive surface electrode.

- **Sacral neuromodulation.** This is inserted into the lower back, and it works on the pelvic nerves. Urogynecologists describe this as a type of pacemaker for the bladder. This procedure can also help improve fecal incontinence if it is present.
- **Surgery.** If nothing else works, there are bladder surgeries that can be helpful for some patients.

Question 9: I have mixed incontinence. What should I consider after conservative treatment options fail?

After trying lifestyle modifications, pelvic-floor muscle exercises, and bladder training, focus on the predominant symptom:

- If your predominant symptom is urge incontinence, use an oral medication or one of the other urge incontinence treatment options.
- If your predominant symptom is stress incontinence, your doctor might recommend a mid-urethral sling. (Sometimes a sling makes the urge incontinence worse. Make sure you discuss this possibility with your doctor before the surgery.)

Question 10: I've been treated for UTIs repeatedly, but I keep having symptoms. Why is that happening?

One possible reason is a condition called *interstitial cystitis* (IC). Interstitial cystitis (aka bladder pain syndrome) is a group of symptoms that include mild to severe bladder pain and an urgent and/or frequent need to urinate. A lot of people with interstitial cystitis are treated repeatedly for urinary tract infections (UTIs), but they don't get better because they don't have an infection. The real problem is interstitial cystitis, which is chronic inflammation of the bladder that causes people to urinate — sometimes painfully — as often as forty to sixty times a day. All patients with IC have bladder pain that is relieved at least partially by urinating. Most, although not all, people with IC do not have urinary leakage (incontinence). If your healthcare practitioner keeps giving you antibiotics even though your urine test never shows a UTI, you might have interstitial cystitis. But this diagnosis should only be made after a thorough workup rules out all other possible causes for your symptoms. It can be treated with oral medication or a number of different medical procedures.

DR. NITA'S NOTE
Advocate for Your Health Like a Pro
When You're Dealing with Urinary Incontinence

Here are some questions to ask your doctor:

1. *Is my diagnosis obvious to you, or do you think I need additional testing?* If your practitioner seems like they don't know what to do next, skip to question 7 below.

2. *Is my incontinence due to a dangerous underlying issue?* Please see page 274 for examples of worrisome signs and symptoms. If your practitioner is concerned about a dangerous underlying issue, make sure they are qualified to assist you. If not, ask to be referred to a specialist. If they are not concerned, move on to question 3 below.

3. *What type of incontinence do I have?* Your doctor might not be able to answer this question at your first

appointment, but if they can't, keep circling back to this question each visit. Remember, we focused on three common types of incontinence in this chapter, but we didn't go into all the possible types.

4. *What are some lifestyle modifications I should make to help my symptoms?* Even if you choose to use medication, I'm a big believer in implementing lifestyle changes to maximize the effectiveness of your treatments.

5. *Do you recommend that I try medication or a particular treatment?* If they do, make sure you understand the risks, benefits, and alternatives.

6. *If my symptoms don't improve in the next six weeks to six months* (you and your doctor will determine how long you'd like to wait)*, what will you recommend next for me?* As you and your doctor try different options, you can keep circling back to this question at the end of each appointment. If you're not happy with your progress, or if your doctor feels like other treatment options are beyond their scope of practice, ask them question 7.

7. *Do you think I need a referral to a specialist?* If you are seeing an internal medicine doctor or a family practice doctor, they might send you to a gynecologist. But know that based on what you need, a gynecologist might recommend that you see a urologist or a urogynecologist. Urologists and urogynecologists, who have extensive training in urinary issues, are more specialized than gynecologists.

Chapter 13

Vulvovaginal TLC

Caring for Your Vulva and Vagina

I get it. You want your vagina and vulva to live up to their full potential. So when you see an advertisement that basically says something like, "Hey, you! Lady with a vagina that smells like a vagina. For a few bucks, I can make your lady parts smell like a field of flowers, fruit, or Chanel No. 5," you think to yourself, "That sounds like an upgrade." But is it really? If your vulva and vagina could talk, if they could tell you what they need to be healthy, happy, and thriving, what would they say?

That's what this chapter is about. When it comes to your vulva and vagina, when are you helping, and when are you self-sabotaging?

VULVOVAGINAL HEALTH CRASH COURSE
What You Need to Know to Patient Like a Pro

Question 1: What's the best way to clean my vagina?
Question 2: Umm. I feel like "doing nothing" is not the right

answer. Won't douching or scented products help (at least a little)?

Question 3: What do you want me to do about my strong vaginal odor, excessive vaginal discharge, or any of the other things that might make me want to douche or use scented products?

Question 4: My doctor keeps telling me my vaginal discharge is due to bacterial vaginosis (BV). What are the symptoms, and why does it keep coming back?

Question 5: How can I get rid of bacterial vaginosis that keeps coming back?

Question 6: What are the risks of untreated bacterial vaginosis?

Question 7: Do you have any tips for recurrent yeast infections?

Question 8: Why am I still having vulvar or vaginal itching even though I've been treated for a yeast infection?

Question 9: What tips do you have for taking care of my vulva?

Question 10: If I only need water (and maybe cleanser) for my vulva, why are there so many fancy feminine hygiene products that promise to clean that area?

Question 1: What's the best way to clean my vagina?

It's really, really hard for people to accept the fact that when it comes to cleaning your vagina, here is what you should do: absolutely nothing. Seriously. Just like tears wash your eyes, your vagina produces a discharge that naturally cleanses it. That means your vagina does not want or need your help when it comes to cleaning. Think of it as a self-cleaning oven.

Question 2: Umm. I feel like "doing nothing" is not the right answer. Won't douching or scented products help (at least a little)?

No. For those of you who aren't familiar with douching, it's when you wash or clean out the vagina. Many douches are sold in stores as prepackaged bags or bottles of water and vinegar, baking soda, or iodine. You squirt the douche upward through a tube or nozzle into your vagina. Then, the water mixture comes back out through your vagina. Some companies try to win you over and say it's fine because it's "medically formulated," or "all natural," but, to be clear, there's nothing you could tell me that would make me say, "Oh, I didn't think about that. Well, in that case you should start douching at home."

Whether you're doing it because of excessive vaginal discharge, vaginal odor, or anything else, douching is a bad idea for a lot of reasons. First of all, it's normal for adult vaginas to have good bacteria and bad bacteria in them. But in a healthy reproductive-age woman's vagina, the good bacteria (called lactobacilli) dominate. And those dominant good bacteria make something called lactic acid to keep your vagina mildly acidic (about the same pH level as tomato juice). That acidity helps to keep the number of bad, disease-causing bacteria in check because they don't thrive in acidic environments. If you douche, it's like you are taking a water hose and washing the good bacteria out of your vagina. That throws your acidic vaginal pH off and allows the bad bacteria to multiply. And that shift in power can lead to bacterial vaginosis, which is an infection that increases your risk of getting STDs, including HIV, if you're exposed. (We will talk more about bacterial vaginosis in later questions.)

Plus, douching also increases the probability that bacteria

will travel up into your uterus and fallopian tubes and around your ovaries (see figure 17). That can cause something called pelvic inflammatory disease (PID), which is a serious infection that can lead to infertility, long-term pelvic pain, or an ectopic pregnancy (which is when a fertilized egg implants and grows outside of the uterus).

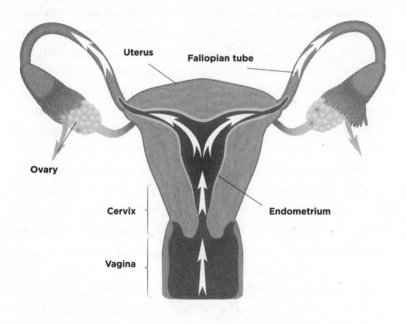

Figure 17. Pelvic inflammatory disease (PID): bacteria ascending into the uterus and fallopian tubes, then spreading around the ovaries

As with douching, using scented products can also decrease the number of good bacteria in your vagina. Scented products can also dehydrate and irritate the vaginal walls. For these reasons and many more, douching and scented products are no good for you or your vagina.

Question 3: What do you want me to do about my strong vaginal odor, excessive vaginal discharge, or any of the other things that might make me want to douche or use scented products?

I want you to see a healthcare practitioner to figure out what's going on. To determine whether your symptoms are due to an underlying issue that needs to be treated, your doctor should do an exam to inspect your vagina and check for infections. Infections can be identified by collecting a small amount of vaginal discharge using a long swab and/or doing a urine test. They may also perform a Pap test, if indicated.

On another note, sometimes what people consider a strong vaginal odor is actually normal. For instance, musky smells are probably just discharge or sweat — yes, it's normal for your vulvovaginal region to have a mild, musky smell. Some women notice a metallic smell during their period. And throughout the month, it's typical to have changes in the amount of discharge you have. So seeing a doctor might help you learn what's normal for your body.

A rotten smell, on the other hand, is frequently a sign that you forgot about a tampon. Those are easy for you or an ob-gyn to remove, but please try not to forget your tampons because toxic shock syndrome — a rare, life-threatening complication — is more likely to happen if a tampon is left in for too long.

Question 4: My doctor keeps telling me my vaginal discharge is due to bacterial vaginosis (BV). What are the symptoms, and why does it keep coming back?

Bacterial vaginosis is the most common cause of abnormal vaginal discharge in women. And I've seen women who have been struggling with it for years and years. So I'm going to get a little more detailed with this answer.

Approximately 50 to 75 percent of women with BV have no symptoms, but if you do develop symptoms, here are some you might experience (all compliments of an overgrowth of the bad bacteria we talked about in question 2):

- A thin white or gray vaginal discharge
- A strong fishlike odor, especially after sex with a man who didn't wear a condom (this is because the bacteria associated with BV create a fishy smell that's amplified when mixed with a man's ejaculate)
- Irritation or itching around the opening of the vagina
- A burning sensation while peeing[1]

We don't know why, but more than half of people who are treated for BV have symptoms again within twelve months. When the BV symptoms come back, it could be because of a reinfection. But more likely the initial infection never completely cleared up because the good bacteria were never able to regain dominance in your vagina.

Here are some things that might be making it hard for you to defeat your bacterial vaginosis infection once and for all:

- **Something called a biofilm is making it hard for you to get rid of the bad bacteria.** A medication can't kill what it can't detect, and unfortunately, sometimes the bad bacteria that cause your BV symptoms are very good at hiding from antibiotics. This is how a biofilm happens: Some forms of bad bacteria are able to stick to your vaginal wall or an item like your copper IUD or progestin IUD.[2] Then bacteria cover themselves with something called a biofilm, which is described by some researchers as an "invisibility cloak" of protection

against antibiotics. Once you're finished with your antibiotic treatment, the bacteria ditch the invisibility cloak
and cause your BV symptoms to recur. Devious, isn't it?
Unfortunately, we don't currently have a commercially
available test to check for biofilms in clinics.

- **Your BV is being caused by bacteria that are
  tougher to kill.** Some types of "bad bacteria" are
  harder to kill than others.
- **Your period.** Blood might provide nutrients that help
  the harmful bacteria thrive. Also, remember that the
  good bacteria like your vagina to be acidic (low pH),
  but your period blood may raise the pH, temporarily
  making your vagina more hospitable to bad bacteria.
  This can especially become an issue if your periods are
  long and/or frequent.
- **Your vaginal microbiome doesn't have enough
  lactobacilli.** Research shows that some women have
  fewer lactobacilli than others, but this isn't because of
  anything you're doing or not doing health-wise.[3]

Other potential factors that increase your risk

- **Having sex.** Many experts believe that women who
  have never had any kind of sex, including receiving
  oral sex, don't get bacterial vaginosis. However, BV isn't
  currently considered a sexually transmitted infection
  because we haven't found a clear disease counterpart
  in males and we haven't identified a single causative
  agent. Here are some theories that may explain what's
  going on.[4] For females with female partners, BV might
  be caused by exposure to the other person's vaginal
  bacteria or biofilm. For females with male partners, the
  increased incidence of BV might be due to the fact
  that semen has a high pH, which makes your vagina

less acidic. Or maybe your partner is transmitting biofilms with BV-causing bacteria.

- **Having sexually transmitted infections.** Having an STI increases the risk of getting BV.
- **Douching.** Women who douche once a week are five times more likely to develop BV than women who don't douche.[5]
- **Smoking cigarettes.** People who smoke have a higher chance of acquiring BV.

Question 5: How can I get rid of bacterial vaginosis that keeps coming back?

If you have BV occasionally, one to seven days of antibiotics will do the trick. But if you have three or more documented symptomatic infections in twelve months, it's time to consider prevention mode. There are different ways to approach recurrent bacterial vaginosis. If a patient has recurrent BV and they haven't tried secnidazole, which is a single-dose oral antibiotic used to treat bacterial vaginosis, I recommend giving that a try. If that doesn't work, or if their insurance won't cover the cost of secnidazole, I typically recommend the following treatment plan for patients who aren't pregnant, planning to become pregnant, or breastfeeding.

Step 1. A seven-day course of one of the following antibiotics:

- ○ **Metronidazole** 500 mg by mouth twice a day for seven days
- ○ **Metronidazole** 0.75 percent gel one applicator full (5 g) into your vagina at bedtime for seven days
- ○ **Clindamycin** 300 mg by mouth twice daily for seven days
- ○ **Clindamycin** 2 percent cream one applicator full (5 g) into your vagina at bedtime for seven days

Step 2. On the same day that you start the antibiotic in step 1, start using boric acid suppositories (600 mg) once daily at bedtime. Continue for thirty days. If you have a biofilm that's protecting the bad bacteria from the antibiotic, boric acid's job is to destroy the biofilm.

Since boric acid is used as a roach killer, some people get a little nervous about this step. But don't worry. I'm not practicing cowboy medicine. This treatment has been studied, and I've seen it work wonders for a lot of women struggling with recurrent BV. Plus, boric acid is also used for many other, less-alarming purposes, including being an ingredient in some eye-washes. If you don't wish to use boric acid, you can skip this step and proceed with the metronidazole gel or clindamycin cream mentioned in step 3. If you do use boric acid, be aware of these precautions:

o *Boric acid can result in death if swallowed!* So keep it away from children, and don't let anyone perform oral sex on you during this treatment.

o You might experience some mild irritation or discharge. Let your doctor know if it's bothersome.

o Your sexual partner might notice skin irritation after exposure to boric acid. If their symptoms are bothersome, they should see a doctor.

o You shouldn't use boric acid if you're pregnant, actively trying to get pregnant, or breastfeeding.

Step 3. One or two days after you finish your treatment, follow up with your doctor. If you're in remission from BV, I recommend metronidazole gel twice weekly for six months. If you can't use metronidazole for some reason, clindamycin cream (2 percent) is an option, but it's less effective and tends to lead to more vaginal yeast infections than metronidazole gel. Clindamycin cream should not be used concurrently with latex condoms. This medication may cause latex to be weakened.

Step 4. After six months of treatment, stop all antibiotics and see how you do.

In addition to taking the medication, here are some tips that may help lower your risk of getting BV again:

- **Practice BV-friendly sex.**
  - ○ Women who have sex with men: Use latex condoms correctly every time you have sex, and avoid spermicide.
  - ○ Women who have sex with women: BV is more common in lesbian women than in heterosexual women. Ask your partner to get tested for bacterial vaginosis and treated if needed. Also, don't share insertive sex toys. Or if you do, cover them with a new condom for each use and clean them after each use.
- **Consider hormonal contraception.** According to some research, hormonal contraception may decrease your risk of BV by making periods lighter.
- **Practice good vulvovaginal hygiene.** Avoid scented soaps and detergents.
- **Watch out for your lube's pH.** Water-based lubricants should have a pH of 3.5 to 4.5. Lubes with a higher pH may increase your odds of BV.
- **Try probiotics.** This is a *maybe*, meaning the jury is still out. But you're free to give them a try. We don't know for sure which strains or combinations of strains are best, and we don't know the optimal dose or duration of use. But if you decide on this option, I recommend choosing one that contains lactobacillus crispatus. Other strains of lactobacillus might also be helpful, such as lactobacillus acidophilus, lactobacillus rhamnosus, and lactobacillus reuteri RC-14. If you use these products, be aware that the quality is frequently poor and the contents are not standardized. (Translation: the products don't always contain what you think they contain.) The FDA also wants consumers to be

aware that patient death has been reported in immunocompromised patients who have used dietary supplements containing live bacteria or yeast.

- **Try Rephresh gel.** Since we don't have well-designed studies to support this suggestion, it's another *maybe*, but you can try using Rephresh gel once weekly and after sex. This gel may help keep your vaginal pH low.
- **Consider the possibility of a biofilm.** If your BV persists in spite of all the suggestions discussed above and your symptoms are bothersome, you can discuss the possibility of an IUD biofilm with your doctor. However, before you remove your very effective birth control, please understand that there is no guarantee that this will solve your recurrent BV problem. So you may be left with no IUD and lingering BV. Because we don't have strong research to support this suggestion, many experts advise against removing IUDs because of recurrent BV. If you decide to remove it, we don't know how long you should wait before replacing the IUD. If you are using anything else that might have a biofilm, such as an Estring (which is a ninety-day vaginal ring used for menopausal changes), consider replacing it before being treated for recurrent BV.

Question 6: What are the risks of untreated bacterial vaginosis?

Asymptomatic BV typically resolves spontaneously over a period of several months. However, you still have these risks even if you don't have any symptoms:

- Having BV increases your risk of getting STDs, such as genital herpes, chlamydia, gonorrhea, and trichomoniasis. It also increases your chances of getting HIV or transmitting it to your partner if you have it.

- Having untreated BV at the time of a transvaginal procedure such as a hysterectomy, pregnancy termination, or a D&C (dilation and curettage) can increase the risk of postoperative infections. For instance, if you have bacterial vaginosis when you have a hysterectomy (removal of your uterus), you have a higher chance of getting an infection of the vaginal cuff (the sewed incision on the top of the vagina that was made during surgery).
- Bacterial vaginosis has been associated with preterm birth. However, despite the association, screening and treating women who don't have symptoms has not been consistently shown to reduce the risk of preterm delivery. Therefore, we don't usually test pregnant people who don't have BV symptoms. But if you have a moderate or high risk of having your baby prematurely, ask your healthcare practitioner if they think you should be checked for BV (even if you don't have symptoms). If you're pregnant and have BV symptoms, you should be treated.

Question 7: Do you have any tips for recurrent yeast infections?

Many women who self-diagnose don't actually have yeast infections, so lab testing may be necessary to confirm that yeast infections are indeed what you're experiencing. Common symptoms of a yeast infection include:

- Itching or irritation of the vulva or vagina
- A burning sensation, especially during urination or sex
- Swelling or redness of the vulva
- Vaginal pain or swelling
- White clumpy (cottage cheese–like) or watery vaginal discharge (though some individuals have no abnormal vaginal discharge)

For occasional yeast infections, an over-the-counter med usually works fine for most people, or your doctor can prescribe a yeast infection cream or an oral pill called fluconazole. But if a patient has been diagnosed with four or more yeast infections in twelve months, that's when I move to prevention mode.

If I have a new patient who is struggling with recurrent yeast infections, the first thing I like to do is determine what I'm up against. To do this, I use a swab to get a sample of vaginal discharge to send to the lab. The lab determines if yeast is a likely cause. If it is, they identify the species of yeast and determine which medication(s) can defeat it. Once we get the results back, one of these three scenarios usually comes into play:

Scenario 1. I learn that the species of yeast causing their symptoms can be treated with our standard "go-to" yeast infection meds, but they need to be treated for a longer period of time. One popular option is to prescribe ten to fourteen days of a topical yeast infection cream, followed by clotrimazole 200 mg vaginal cream twice weekly for six months. (If you'd prefer something oral, you can opt for fluconazole 150 mg every 72 hours for three doses, followed by maintenance with fluconazole 150 mg by mouth once a week for six months.) If the yeast infection comes back after we stop the six-month treatment course, some patients resume the weekly medication for months or years.

Scenario 2. I find out that their infection is due to yeast that is resistant to standard "go-to" yeast infection meds discussed in scenario 1. Discussing all the treatment recommendations goes beyond the scope of this crash course, but if you have recurrent yeast infections, ask your doctor if they are sure the med they are prescribing is the best option for the species of yeast causing your infection. For example, the meds ibrexafungerp or oteseconazole work well for some resistant yeast infections. (Note: some species of yeasts can form the same type of biofilm that we discussed in question 4.)

Scenario 3. I determine that their itching isn't due to yeast. See question 8 for more on this.

If someone has recurrent vaginal yeast infections, I check them for diabetes. And, if they are at high risk, I also check them for HIV or AIDS.

Question 8: Why am I still having vulvar or vaginal itching even though I've been treated for a yeast infection?

Not all vulvovaginal itches are due to yeast. So if your itching doesn't resolve with treatment, ask your doctor if something else might be going on. Here are some other possible causes:

Contact dermatitis is a reaction to a product that results in an itchy rash. I see this a lot. The culprit can be anything from a new soap to underwear, tampons, sanitary pads, douches, scented sprays, vulva masks, vaginal steaming, lubricants, condoms, or toilet paper. New exposure to an allergen is most likely to induce a reaction, but it is also possible to develop an allergy to a product you've been using for years.

Hormonal changes that come with perimenopause or menopause can result in itching due to vulvar and vaginal dryness. Your healthcare practitioner may suggest an over-the-counter vaginal moisturizer or a prescription local vaginal estrogen cream, ring, or vaginal insert.

Infections such as bacterial vaginosis or sexually transmitted infections can also lead to itching.

Skin conditions such as *lichen sclerosus*, which is characterized by white, patchy vulvar skin, are another possible reason. A biopsy may be helpful if your practitioner suspects a skin condition like lichen sclerosus but they are not sure of the diagnosis.

Vulvar cancer or precancer may cause vulvar itching as well as burning or bleeding. Other symptoms include vulvar skin sores, rashes, or warts that don't go away, or changes in the color of your vulvar skin. If there is any suspicion of cancer or precancer, a vulvar biopsy is definitely indicated.

Question 9: What tips do you have for taking care of my vulva?

- Don't believe people who tell you that a vulva-cleansing product will restore your vaginal pH. Your vaginal pH and vulvar pH are two separate issues. Trying to use a vulvar product to cure a vaginal infection is like thinking you can make your breath smell better by using toothpaste to wash your face. It ain't gonna happen. (And using these products inside the vagina will increase your chance of getting a vaginal infection, like bacterial vaginosis. So please don't do that either.)

- Less is more. My top choice for cleaning the vulva is plain warm water. I'm a huge fan of bidets. However, I also understand that some vulvas are more tolerant than others. So if you use a particular product on your vulva and you don't experience any issues, then it's OK if you continue using that product. (But don't forget that your vulva is not your vagina. My recommendation is to let your vaginal discharge do all the work for vaginal cleaning.)

- There's an exception to my water-only rule. If you have fecal or urinary incontinence, chronic exposure to urine or feces can irritate your skin. Therefore, if your skin can tolerate something "stronger," I recommend a cleanser that has a pH between 5.0 and 7.0, such as Eucerin pH5. And if you need something when you're not at home, you can use an unscented wipe. If you want something stronger than water because you are on your period or because you are sweating a lot, I still recommend the same options.

- Your vulva might need to be moisturized. If things like skin irritation from pubic hair removal, soaps, or wipes leave your vulvar skin feeling dry and/or itchy, you can stop doing things that are drying out your skin (when that's a possibility), or you can try a vulvar moisturizer. There are lots of great options, but my vulvar moisturizers of choice are coconut oil, hyaluronic acid moisturizers, or any diaper rash ointment or cream. But whenever trying any new topical product, you should try it on a small test area to make sure it doesn't irritate your skin. And you should only try one new option at a time. Note: Products that contain oil will weaken latex condoms.
- Be careful with hair removal. As far as your vulvar hair goes, whether you want to rock a bush, go bare, leave a landing strip, or profess your love by shaving your partner's initials down below, your vulvar "hairdo" is your business. Just please be careful, especially if you have a medical condition like diabetes that increases your risk of infection. I've seen some people in the hospital with a serious abscess after what seemed like a simple shaving or waxing nick.

DR. NITA'S NOTE
Don't Neglect Your Hood

Just like under the foreskin of the penis, a woman can accumulate a thick white or yellow deposit called smegma — a combination of oily secretions and dead skin — under her clitoral hood or in the folds of the labia. Freshly formed smegma is not a problem, but stale, accumulated smegma is. If it builds up, the oil and dead skin will mix together to create an ideal breeding ground for bad-smelling bacteria. Sometimes it kinda smells like sour milk or Swiss cheese. Plus, the built-up smegma can cause clitoral adhesions that make clitoral stimulation painful. So be sure to keep this part of your vulva clean by gently washing it.

Question 10: If I only need water (and maybe cleanser) for my vulva, why are there so many fancy feminine hygiene products that promise to clean that area?

Because big companies like money.

DR. NITA'S NOTE
Advocate for Your Health Like a Pro
When You Have Vaginal or Vulvar Complaints

Here are some questions to ask your doctor:

1. *May I have an exam?* A physical exam can give us a lot of information. If you go to an appointment because of vaginal discharge, itching, or odor, ask to be examined.
2. *What do you think is causing my symptoms?* Unless you are 100 percent sure you haven't been exposed to a sexually transmitted infection (STI), I strongly recommend that you get screened for STIs.

3. *Were you able to rule out anything today?* When it comes to vaginal discharge, some tests can be done in-office, and others are sent to an outside lab.

4. *When will I get my results?* Ask this question if you have labs that were sent off. In most cases, results will be posted online. If you don't have access to your electronic record for some reason, make sure someone notifies you of your results. Do away with the no-news-is-good-news mentality.

5. If you presented with vulvar itching and they say, "don't worry about it," or they give you a steroid cream, ask, *How long will it take for the itching to totally resolve?* If you have persistent itching and they don't know the cause, a biopsy might provide additional information. If you are diagnosed with a skin condition, make sure you ask if that condition increases your risk of certain cancers. For example, people with untreated lichen sclerosus have an increased risk of developing vulvar cancer.

Pro tips

- If you are diagnosed with an STI, ask if you need to follow up for repeat testing. If you do, ask when.
- If you get tested before the window period (see page 87 if you are not familiar with this term), ask when you should follow up for repeat testing.

Chapter 14

When Your Hormones Go Off a Cliff

Menopause

A few years ago, I made plans to go to a fancy party with a friend of mine who was in her late thirties. Since she was a mom with three small kids, a husband, a demanding job, two dogs, and an interestingly rebellious gerbil, this was a big deal for her. We'd been planning this girls' night out for weeks.

When we arrived, my friend looked fantastic. And I'm not talking about an ordinary kind of fantastic: she looked like she had stepped off the cover of *Vogue*. About two hours into the event, she excused herself to the bathroom, which (of course) wasn't a big deal. But little did I know, that trip to the bathroom was the beginning of the end of our magnificent night. Y'all, when she got back, it looked like she had gone to the gym. Her mascara was running, her hair was sticking to her forehead and the back of her neck, and her silk shirt was sticking to her chest. Of course, at that point I said, "Let's head out." And her response as she looked at me through her glasses that were starting to fog up was, "Great idea."

On the way home, the only thing she said was, "It feels like a fire-breathing dragon is living in my body. I don't want to talk about it right now."

That was one point for the menopause transition.

Many twenty-, thirty-, and even forty-something-year-olds think menopause is something that suddenly appears in a woman's late forties or sometimes in her fifties, but that's not how the story always unfolds. It's true that the average age of menopause in the US is 51.4, but you may notice changes as your body starts making the transition into menopause years before then. During this period, which is known as the menopause transition, the climacteric, or perimenopause, the amount of estrogen produced by the ovaries begins to fluctuate. As a result, you may start to experience classic menopause symptoms like hot flashes or vaginal dryness. Your periods may also become irregular, or they might start coming closer together or further apart. Or you may also notice that your periods become heavier or lighter. (Note: You should always tell your doctor about menstrual changes, since they could be a sign of something else.)

The menopause transition (and menopause) has lots of symptoms. However, since hot flashes and vaginal dryness are the major complaints, impacting up to 82 and 85 percent of females in the United States, respectively, those are the issues that I will focus on in this chapter. If you are looking for an accessible, thorough book about menopause, I highly recommend *The Menopause Book* by Pat Wingert and Barbara Kantrowitz, *The Menopause Manifesto* by Dr. Jen Gunter, or Dr. Lauren Streicher's *Inside Information* book series. Also, if you are looking for a local menopause guru to help you out, go to the North American Menopause Society's (NAMS) website (menopause.org) and plug in your zip code to get a list of qualified practitioners. Why? One day, Dr. Mary Jane Minkin, founder of madameovary.com, jokingly told me that she and some other practitioners from the NAMS call themselves the

Menopause Mafia. That's how serious these practitioners are about demolishing menopause symptoms!

MENOPAUSE CRASH COURSE
What You Need to Know to Patient Like a Pro

Question 1: What is menopause?

Question 2: Why does menopause happen?

Question 3: Which tests will let me know if I'm perimeno-pausal, and once I'm perimenopausal or menopausal, what symptoms will I experience?

Question 4: How can I treat hot flashes without using hor-mones?

Question 5: What about vitamins, supplements, herbal rem-edies, and other alternative options?

Question 6: My hot flashes are kicking my butt. I really want to take hormones, but why do people say they're dan-gerous?

Question 7: Should I get a blood, urine, or saliva test to check my hormone levels to customize my hormone doses?

Question 8: Are compounded hormones safer?

Question 9: Have compounded bioidentical hormones been proven to be safer than commercially produced bioiden-tical hormones?

Question 10: What can I do about signs and symptoms of genitourinary syndrome of menopause (GSM)?

Question 1: What is menopause?

Menopause is defined as the time in a woman's life when the ovaries stop producing estrogen and menstrual periods per-manently stop. After menopause, a woman can no longer get pregnant.

Question 2: Why does menopause happen?

Before menopause, your ovaries make most of your estrogen. And that estrogen travels all over your body, where it does things like help prevent vaginal dryness and keep you hot flash–free. Once your ovaries wind down their estrogen production, you might start to notice symptoms of menopause. There are two ways that people lose their ovarian estrogen supply:[1]

- **Natural menopause.** Natural menopause is diagnosed after a woman hasn't had a period for twelve consecutive months without any other explanation. This type of menopause usually happens between the ages of 40 and 58, with the average age being 51.4. But, although 95 percent of women are menopausal by age 56, a few women don't reach menopause until they are in their sixties. Genetics play a big role in determining at what age you'll go through menopause, but your lifestyle and environmental factors are also very important. For instance, smoking can cause menopause to come one to two years earlier — just in case you needed another reason to ditch your ridiculously expensive cancer-, stroke-, and heart attack-causing cigarettes.
- **Induced menopause.** This type of menopause, which can happen any time after puberty, occurs because an outside force, like chemotherapy, radiation or surgical removal of both your ovaries causes you to lose the estrogen that was being produced by your ovaries. Of note, when you suddenly lose your estrogen supply (like you do with surgical removal of both ovaries), you are more likely to experience menopausal symptoms such as hot flashes.

If natural or induced menopause occurs before the age of forty, it's called *premature menopause*, and if either happens between the ages of forty and forty-five, it's called *early menopause*. Premature or early menopause may result in a higher risk of health problems such as heart disease and osteoporosis; however, proper treatment can lower that risk.

Question 3: Which tests will let me know if I'm perimenopausal, and once I'm perimenopausal or menopausal, what symptoms will I experience?

Many people who believe they are perimenopausal ask for a blood test to confirm the diagnosis. When someone makes this request, clinicians typically check their levels of follicle-stimulating hormone (FSH) and estradiol. However, these blood tests have limitations.

FSH is a hormone produced by the pituitary gland, which is located at the base of the brain. FSH travels to the ovaries and stimulates the ovaries to produce the hormone estradiol, which is a potent estrogen. In postmenopausal women, FSH is consistently high and estradiol is consistently low. The problem with checking these labs in perimenopause is that FSH and estrogen levels rise and fall unpredictably. For example, during perimenopause your FSH may be high on Monday, low on Wednesday, and high again on Thursday. Therefore, even if your doctor recommends repeat blood draws (that are at least two weeks apart, for example), due to the unpredictability of your levels, that won't necessarily give you a definitive diagnosis. So, in summary, you can have normal labs and still be perimenopausal. Furthermore, if you are taking a birth control pill that has estrogen, the lab test won't be accurate because the estrogen in the birth control will impact your lab values.

Instead of relying on labs to diagnose perimenopause, clinicians typically consider your age and any symptoms you may have, which brings us to the second part of the question: What types of changes might you notice during perimenopause/menopause?

Some people never notice any symptoms, not even a single hot flash. Their period disappears one day, and that's it for them. But when people have symptoms, menopause can affect them from head to toe. Here are some ways it might pop up in your life:[2]

Adult acne
Anger
Anxiety
Bloating
Bone loss
Brain fog/memory
  problems
Breast tenderness
Chills
Constipation
Decreased libido
Depression
Difficulty concentrating
Dizziness
Dry skin and hair
Dysuria (pain, discomfort, or
  burning when you pee)
Fatigue
Headaches
Heart palpitations
Heavier periods
Hot flashes
Irregular periods
Irritability
Itchy skin
Joint and muscle aches

Lighter periods
Menstrual migraines
Missed periods
Mood swings (laughing one
  minute and crying the
  next)
Muscle tension and
  aches
Nervousness
New-onset snoring
Night sweats
Painful sex
Panic attacks
Recurrent UTIs
Restless leg syndrome
Sleep problems
Stress urinary inconti-
  nence
Thinning hair and dry
  skin
Urinary frequency
Urinary urgency
Weight gain and slowed
  metabolism
Worry
Vaginal dryness

Periods that are heavy or irregular always need to be evaluated. Even though it might be because of the hormonal changes associated with perimenopause, you need to make sure another cause (such as fibroids or endometrial cancer/precancer) isn't the culprit. See chapter 9 to learn more about the possible reasons for heavy, irregular periods.

DR. NITA'S NOTE
Is It Hot in Here, or Is It Just Me?

A hot flash is a sudden sensation of extreme heat in the upper body, particularly the face, neck, and chest. We aren't certain why they happen, but here's one theory: In a premenopausal woman, the body's thermostat (hypothalamus) springs into action to cool her body down if her core body temperature increases by 0.4°C. But for unknown reasons, when a woman's estrogen drops in menopause or in the menopause transition, the thermostat no longer tolerates a 0.4°C temperature increase. Instead, when your estrogen-deprived thermostat notices a slight change, it decides to "help you out" by giving you a hot flash, which is a chain of events intended to cool your body down.

The warm feeling happens because of inappropriate dilation of some blood vessels along with increased skin blood flow. The sweating you experience is your body's way of getting rid of heat quickly to bring your core body temperature down. Then shivering may occur if your body needs to get your core temperature back up to normal. In other words, not only does your body unnecessarily make you sweat to cool down, but it sometimes overshoots and makes your temp drop more than needed so you have to shiver to warm yourself up again. Hormone therapy works because it makes your thermostat go back to the way it functioned when you were premenopausal.[3]

Hot flashes hit some people a lot harder than others. They might be mild, or you might feel like your body could melt a sheet of ice. Some people average less than one hot flash a day, and others have one an hour, day and night. They usually last one to five minutes, but they can last as long as thirty. On average, women experience hot flashes for five to ten years, but some women have them for much longer. According to some research, African American women tend to get hit the longest and the hardest. (Yay for me!)

Question 4: How can I treat hot flashes without using hormones?

Estrogen is the most effective hot flash treatment option, but here are some other things you can consider.

Medicine-free options

- **Try cognitive behavioral therapy (CBT).** This treatment, which is a structured type of talk therapy done with a therapist alone or in groups, teaches you to separate physical experiences from your feelings and thoughts. According to research, menopausal women trained in CBT reported a 65 to 78 percent decrease in complaints about their hot flashes.[4]
- **Consider clinical hypnosis.** This option, which combines working with a hypnosis practitioner and incorporating at-home activities, focuses on increasing your level of relaxation. There's limited data on this, but you can give it a try.
- **Know your triggers.** Hot flashes can be brought on by excessive alcohol, cigarettes, spicy food, sugar, caffeine, stress, or hot weather. To figure out what's triggering your hot flashes, write down when you have a hot flash and what you were doing before it happened to see if there is a pattern.

- **Maintain a healthy body weight.** Obesity is a risk factor for hot flashes. We are not sure why this is the case, but some researchers believe it's because adipose (fat) tissue functions as an insulator, trapping the heat.
- **Respect your sensitive thermostat.** Dress in layers of clothing that can be easily shed, lower the room temperature, use fans, and try to have ice cold water available to drink in case you get a hot flash.
- **Try electroacupuncture.** During this procedure, pulses of weak electrical current are sent through acupuncture needles into acupuncture points in the skin. I'd like to see more studies confirming that this works, but some women report relief.
- **Find DIY ways to relax.** I don't have sound scientific proof that yoga, for example, will demolish your hot flashes, but some women swear by it. If you find that easily accessible DIY relaxation techniques work for you, that's great!

Nonhormonal options that may work

Of these five options, the SSRI paroxetine (7.5 mg/day) is the only nonhormonal therapy that is approved by the FDA for the treatment of hot flashes in the United States.

- **Antidepressants.** Selective serotonin reuptake inhibitors (SSRIs) and selective norepinephrine reuptake inhibitors (SNRIs). Low-dose antidepressants have been shown to help hot flashes in women, even if they are not depressed. Examples of antidepressants that may help you out include:
  - **SSRIs:** paroxetine 7.5 mg/day, citalopram 10–20 mg/day, and escitalopram 10–20 mg/day
  - **SNRI:** venlafaxine 75 mg/day
  Note: Some of these medications may impact your

sexual desire, arousal, or ability to orgasm. These side effects are reversible, but to decrease the probability of them, start with the lowest possible dose and slowly increase it every eight to twelve weeks.

- **Antiseizure medication.** Gabapentin is one antiseizure medication that is effective for treating hot flashes in some women, even if they don't have seizures. While this option can be used for hot flashes that occur during the day, it tends to be particularly helpful for women who mainly struggle with hot flashes at night (aka night sweats). A single dose of gabapentin one hour before bedtime may resolve the flashes that wake you up at night. Or, if they do wake you, you might have an easier time falling asleep again. If you are using the medication for night sweats, you can start at 100 mg one hour before bedtime. Then, if your hot flashes persist, your practitioner can increase the dosage to a maximum of 900 mg. (However, medication side effects frequently limit what dose women can tolerate.) Pregabalin 150–300 mg daily is another option, but it hasn't been studied as extensively as gabapentin.
- **Anticholinergic medication.** A medication named oxybutynin, which is frequently used for urinary problems caused by overactive bladder, may also help with hot flashes. The optimal daily dose for hot flashes appears to be 5 to 10 mg by mouth. However, studies suggest that taking this medication for more than a few months increases the risk of dementia later in life. In one study that involved over 300,000 adults, the risk of dementia increased by approximately 50 percent in adults over fifty-five who took a daily anticholinergic for at least three years.
- **Antihypertensive medication.** The blood pressure medication clonidine (0.1 mg/day) is another option. But it's not frequently used because of its side effect

profile, which includes dry mouth, dizziness, constipation, and sedation.

- **Stellate-ganglion block.** Some preliminary data suggest that local injection of anesthetic into the stellate ganglion (a group of nerves in the neck) may reduce hot flashes in women with contraindications to hormone therapy. However, additional studies are needed to assess the safety and effectiveness of this technique.

Question 5: What about vitamins, supplements, herbal remedies, and other alternative options?

My "sure, give it a try" list:

- Relizen is a pollen extract that many women find helpful when it comes to hot flashes. It takes around three months to fully kick in.
- Phytoestrogens are plant derived substances with estrogenic biologic activity. Examples include the isoflavones genistein and daidzein, which are found in high amounts in soybeans, soy products, and red clover. These natural compounds haven't consistently been shown to help hot flashes, but this option appears to be safe. Many people have reported the most relief with S-equol, which is a derivative of daidzein. (Note: Most experts agree that dietary soy is safe in women with estrogen receptor positive breast cancer, but some believe that dietary supplements should be avoided until their safety has been established.)

My "I'd pass" list:

- Vitamin E 800 international units (IU) a day was shown to result in one less hot flash a day. However, taking 400 IU or more of vitamin E per day is associated with an increased risk of mortality. Therefore, I don't recommend this option.

- Black cohosh is commonly used, but liver toxicity has been reported and data are conflicting regarding effectiveness. So it's on my pass list for now.

- This list is not all-inclusive, but here are some other therapies that haven't been proven to be more effective than placebo (a placebo is a harmless pill, medicine, or procedure that is prescribed for psychological benefit only): evening primrose oil, ginseng, dong quai, wild yam and progesterone creams, reflexology, and magnetic devices. Why is it that some people swear these options work? They may be experiencing the placebo effect. In hot flash studies where people are given a placebo, up to 50 percent of them will say their hot flashes decreased. In other words, just thinking you're taking medicine that will help your hot flashes makes you feel better. In addition to not having studies to prove that they work, some herbal remedies and supplements have serious safety concerns.

I look forward to having more well-designed studies that prove the safety and effectiveness of more of these options. In the meantime, I recommend that you proceed with caution. After considering your personal history, your practitioner may recommend options such as vitamins, supplements, or herbal remedies, but I just want to make sure you understand the risks first.

Question 6: My hot flashes are kicking my butt. I really want to take hormones, but why do people say they're dangerous?

Menopausal hormone therapy (MHT) was very popular. Then, this happened: In the 1990s approximately 27,000 menopausal women between fifty and seventy-nine joined a study called the Women's Health Initiative. In this study, which was trying to determine if hormone therapy impacted a woman's risk of heart disease, some of the women in the study were given estrogen and some were given estrogen and progestin. The reason that some women got progestin is that if you still have a uterus, you need to take progestin along with the estrogen to prevent cancer of the endometrium (the inside lining of the uterus). If you don't have a uterus, you can take estrogen alone. These were the results of the study:

Table 9. Women's Health Initiative Study Findings for All Ages (50–79)[5]

	Estrogen	Estrogen and progestin
Breast cancer	Varies; reduces risk in some women	Increased risk
Heart disease	No change in risk	Increased risk
Stroke	Increased risk	Increased risk
Blood clots	Increased risk	Increased risk
Bone health	Decreased risk of fractures	Decreased risk of fractures
Colon cancer	No change in risk	Decreased risk

After seeing these results, people freaked out. And a lot of women said, "Nope. No more hormones for me!" But ... here's one problem with the interpretation of the study: The study results listed above aren't an accurate representation of the typical women who request menopausal hormone therapy. The average study participant's age was sixty-three. However, almost all women who seek initiation of medical therapy for menopausal symptoms do so in their late forties or fifties. For healthy women in this age group, the absolute risk of complications for women taking MHT for five years is very low. To put things in perspective, here are the numbers for women in their fifties:

Table 10. Women's Health Initiative Study Findings for Ages 50–59[6]

Number of cases per 10,000 women per year				
	Estrogen	Placebo	Estrogen plus progestin	Placebo
Breast cancer	21	29	31	26
Heart disease	17	27	22	17
Stroke	16	16	14	10
Blood clots	15	13	19	8
Hip fracture	4	1	1	3
Colorectal cancer	7	12	4	5

We now know that women who start hormone therapy at an older age or farther past menopause have an increased risk of adverse events. Therefore, we currently recommend that women start menopausal hormone therapy before the age of sixty or within ten years of becoming menopausal. We also tell women to take the appropriate dose for the appropriate duration.

Going into detail about medication selection goes beyond

the scope of this book, but the books I recommended earlier (*The Menopause Book* by Pat Wingert and Barbara Kantrowitz, *The Menopause Manifesto* by Dr. Jen Gunter, or *Hot Flash Hell* from the *Inside Information* book series by Dr. Lauren Streicher) will tell you everything you could possibly want to know. In the meantime, here are some fundamentals:

- **Estrogen tips.** You can get prescription estrogen in pills or a vaginal ring that delivers estrogen to the whole body (this dose is higher than the one you'd use if your only symptom was vaginal dryness). Prescription estrogen can also be absorbed through your skin via gels, patches, sprays, and emulsions. A lot of doctors prefer nonpill forms of estrogen because the risk of blood clots is lower with those forms.
- **Progesterone tips.** If you still have a uterus and need progesterone to go along with your estrogen, progesterone comes in a pill form, a patch, or a device that's placed in the uterus. (Some clinicians recommend a progesterone cream. However, at this time we don't have the research needed to prove that any available progesterone creams are reliably absorbed through the skin to protect you from endometrial cancer. Therefore, if you need to add progesterone to your estrogen in order to protect your uterus from endometrial cancer, I do not recommend using progesterone cream.)

According to some experts, women who have any of the following should consider an alternative to hormones:

- History of breast cancer
- Coronary heart disease

- History of blood clots
- Stroke
- Active liver disease
- Unexplained vaginal bleeding
- High risk for endometrial cancer
- History of transient ischemic attack (TIA; also called a mini-stroke)

Note: Standard menopausal hormone therapy, which has a much lower dose of estrogen than combined estrogen-progestin contraceptives, does not provide effective contraception. Therefore, if you need birth control and you desire treatment for hot flashes while you are in your thirties or forties, your clinician might recommend a low-dose combined estrogen-progestin oral contraceptive pill. If you still desire treatment for hot flashes in your early to mid-fifties, they might recommend switching to menopausal hormone therapy.

If you decide to stop birth control and you don't wish to transition to menopausal hormone therapy, consider tapering the oral contraceptive by one pill per week. This will help decrease the probability of hot flashes, which are common when women who are around fifty years old stop taking estrogen abruptly.

Question 7: Should I get a blood, urine, or saliva test to check my hormone levels to customize my hormone doses?

No. Those tests have not been proven to work. The American College of Obstetricians and Gynecologists (ACOG) states, "Despite claims to the contrary, evidence is inadequate to support increased efficacy or safety for individualized hormone therapy regimens based on salivary, serum, or urinary testing."[7] The best method is to start low and slowly increase the dose until your symptoms resolve.

Question 8: Are compounded hormones safer?

No. Compounded hormones are custom-made products that have been tailored to a specific patient's needs based on a physician's prescription. The prescription dosing is frequently based on the unreliable salivary, serum, or urine testing we discussed in question 7. Furthermore, compounding pharmacies, which is where the compounded hormones are made, usually receive less scrutiny, so the dose prescribed might not match what you actually get. (Translation: They don't always use the ingredients they say they used. In some cases, the dose of hormones and the overall purity can vary from batch to batch.)

Question 9: Have compounded bioidentical hormones been proven to be safer than commercially produced bioidentical hormones?

No. *Bioidentical* means that the hormones used for therapy are identical in molecular structure to the hormones produced by the ovaries. Bioidentical hormones include commercially available products that are approved by the FDA, such as estradiol and micronized progesterone, as well as compounded preparations that are not regulated by the FDA. Although compounded bioidentical hormones are marketed as being safer than commercial bioidentical hormones, that claim isn't backed by sound scientific research.

If you are going to use bioidentical hormones, please make sure they are commercial products that are approved by the FDA. When drugs are FDA approved, they are required to pass tests that prove that they are safe and effective.

Question 10: What can I do about signs and symptoms of genitourinary syndrome of menopause (GSM)?

GSM refers to all the ways that menopause impacts your vagina, vulva, and lower urinary tract. GSM symptoms can include:

- discomfort with intercourse
- decreased vaginal lubrication during sexual activity
- vulvar and vaginal dryness
- vaginal burning
- vaginal discharge
- genital itching
- decreased vaginal elasticity
- shortening of the vaginal canal
- burning with urination
- urinary urgency
- urinary frequency
- urinary incontinence
- recurrent UTIs

Treatment

First-line therapy for GSM includes hormone-free vaginal moisturizers and lubricants.

The vaginal moisturizer, which doesn't require a prescription, must be consistently used two to three times a week (even if you are not planning to have sex soon). Vaginal moisturizers help your vaginal tissue trap moisture and make your tissue thicker and more elastic. As a result, they provide long-term relief for vaginal dryness, and they reduce vaginal itching, irritation, and pain with sex. Two excellent options include Replens Long-Lasting Vaginal Moisturizer or products with hyaluronic acid in them (e.g., Revaree Hyaluronic Acid suppositories).

However, since these moisturizers aren't typically covered by insurance, they can be pricey.

In addition to the moisturizer, you should also use a vaginal lubricant each time you have intercourse. Unlike a moisturizer, the lubricant won't change your vaginal tissue, but lube is still important because it will decrease friction during sex. Categories of lube include water-based, silicone, hybrid (water and silicone), and oil-based. Here are some lube selection tips, which you should use even if you aren't peri- or postmenopausal.

- **Water-based lubes.** When it comes to water-based lubricants, you want one that has a pH and osmolality that are close to the pH and osmolality of your vaginal secretions. (pH refers to the level of acidity, and osmolality refers to the concentration of molecules in water. If something has a high osmolality, it has a lot of molecules. If it has a low osmolality it has fewer molecules.) This translates into you looking for a water-based lube with a pH of 3.5 to 4.5 and an osmolality close to 300 mOsm/kg.

  Most lubes have a "vaginal-friendly pH," but an appropriate osmolality can be harder to come by. Ideally, you want the osmolality to be around 300 mOsm/kg (like your vaginal secretions), but you definitely never want it to be over 1,200 mOsm/kg. The higher the osmolality, the higher the probability that the lube will pull water out of your vaginal tissue, causing vaginal dryness and irritation. Not only is this counterproductive for sex, but the dryness also increases the chances of you getting microtears during penetration which then increases your risk of acquiring a sexually transmitted infection if you are exposed. A couple of good water-based lubricant options include Good Clean Love and Pulse H2Oh!

- **Silicone lubes.** This type of lube tends to be more

expensive, but a little silicone lubricant goes a long way. This type is very slippery and adheres to the tissue longer than water-based lubes. And it's very unlikely to cause an allergic reaction. Also, you don't have to worry about pH or osmolality issues (they are not a factor with silicone-based lube). One important downside is that this type of lube should not be placed directly on some silicone toys because it may break down the surface of the toy. If you have a silicone toy, either use a water-based lube or put a condom on the toy when using silicone lubricant.

- **Oil-based lubes.** Cooking oils such as olive oil or coconut oil are examples of options that fall in this category. Many women do fine with cooking oil, but if you happen to notice an increased frequency of yeast infections, try using a different type of lubricant. Unlike water-based and silicone lubricants, oil-based lubricants are not compatible with latex condoms because they increase the risk of condom breakage.

If your symptoms don't go away with moisturizers and lubricants, your doctor may recommend vaginal estrogen in the form of a cream, tablet, gel, or ring. Other options include an oral medication called ospemifene or vaginal DHEA. In addition to helping vaginal dryness, prescription medication may also alleviate urinary symptoms such as recurrent urinary tract infections or urinary urgency.

Laser therapy has shown promise in a research setting, especially in the population of breast cancer survivors who may be hesitant to pursue hormonal therapy and often have more severe vaginal dryness. This option, which is not typically covered by insurance, tends to be very expensive. Some clinicians swear by the results, and I have spoken to patients who report a benefit after laser therapy. However, some experts feel that additional research is needed before this recommendation can be made.

Also, remember that things that didn't irritate you in the past may irritate you now. So less is more! Watch out for scented soaps, detergents, and flavored, warming, or cooling lubes.

DR. NITA'S NOTE
Advocate for Your Health Like a Pro When Dealing with Menopausal Symptoms

Here are some questions to ask your doctor:

Hot Flashes

1. *Do you think my hot flashes are because of low estrogen, or is something else going on?* If you are in your late forties with irregular periods, the menopause transition is probably the culprit. However, there are other reasons for hot flashes, such as diabetes, thyroid issues, anxiety, or excessive alcohol. By assessing your history, performing a physical exam, and drawing some labs (if needed), your doctor can determine if a nonmenopause issue might be the problem.

2. *Do you think my hot flashes can be controlled with lifestyle modifications or a safe nonhormonal treatment option? If so, which one(s)?* As discussed earlier, menopausal hormone therapy is safe for appropriately selected patients. However, whether you're inquiring about menopause treatment or anything else related to your health, it is crucial that you know about all your treatment options.

3. *Based on my personal history and family history, am I a good candidate for menopausal hormone therapy?* If the answer is no, remember that there are other available options.

4. *If I use hormones, which mode of delivery do you think is safest for me?* This is where your doctor's expertise will come into play. Not all ob-gyns get a lot of training about menopause treatments. If your doctor seems unsure and you don't know where to turn, you can search for a practitioner on menopause.org. If you can't find a local practitioner and your insurance will cover the cost, consider scheduling a telemedicine appointment with a menopause specialist who doesn't practice medicine close by.

5. *What are the risks of taking hormone therapy?* As with any medication, it's important to weigh the risks and the benefits.

Vaginal Dryness

1. *Do you think my symptoms are due to low estrogen? If so, will vaginal moisturizers or lubricants help?* To determine if your symptoms are due to low estrogen, your clinician should perform a physical exam. If they recommend vaginal moisturizers and lubricants but those don't provide relief, ask for another treatment, such as vaginal estrogen, at your follow-up appointment. Also, if you are concerned about a vaginal infection at any point, make sure you let your doctor know so they can run the appropriate tests.

2. *I like to use* (insert the name of your lube and moisturizer of choice). *Are these good options for me?* Your

goal is to make sure you aren't using something that is likely to cause vaginal irritation or dryness.

Other Health Considerations

1. *What else should I be doing to take care of my health during the menopause transition?* This chapter focused on hot flashes and vaginal dryness, but as you know, there is a lot more to consider when it comes to your health. Your doctor should be able to tailor your recommendations based on your personal and family history.

2. *Should I be taking calcium and vitamin D supplements? If so, at what dosage?* After age thirty-five, a small amount of bone loss is normal for men and women. But during menopause, women lose bone more rapidly due to the decreased level of estrogen. If you lose too much bone, that will increase the risk of osteoporosis, and osteoporosis increases the risk of bone fractures. Make sure you stay up to date with your bone mineral density scans — these usually start at age sixty-five, but some people need them earlier. Also, make sure you are doing weight-bearing exercises.

3. *Can you calculate my fracture risk?* The fracture risk assessment tool (FRAX) is a computer program that helps predict the risk of having a fracture within the next ten years in women forty to ninety years of age who are not taking prescription osteoporosis drugs.

Chapter 15

A Silent Sisterhood

Miscarriages and Infertility

Worldwide there are approximately forty-four pregnancy losses each *minute*. That means that today alone approximately 63,360 women will miscarry.[1] (For this calculation, *miscarriage* is defined as a pregnancy loss before the baby can live outside the womb.) Infertility is also common, impacting 48 million couples around the world. Yet many of the individuals who are affected by pregnancy loss or infertility feel alone.

If you are experiencing infertility or miscarriages, or you're trying to support someone who's dealing with these issues, this chapter is for you.

INFERTILITY AND MISCARRIAGE CRASH COURSE
What You Need to Know to Patient Like a Pro

Infertility

Question 1: What is the official definition of *infertility*?

Question 2: If I'm a uterus owner, when should I consider an infertility workup?

Question 3: Why can't I get pregnant?

Question 4: What are some common reasons for these steps to be disrupted?

Question 5: If I need a workup, what would it involve?

Question 6: What are the treatment options?

Pregnancy Loss

Question 7: What causes a miscarriage?

Question 8: What's the likelihood of having another miscarriage?

Question 9: Will trying again too soon increase my chance of another miscarriage?

Infertility and Miscarriages

Question 10: What can I do to increase my chances of getting pregnant if I have infertility or if I'm trying to get pregnant after having a miscarriage?

Infertility

Question 1: What is the official definition of *infertility*?

For women under thirty-five, *infertility* is defined as not being able to get pregnant after having unprotected sex or donor insemination for one year. If a woman is thirty-five or older, infertility is defined as not being able to get pregnant after having unprotected sex or donor insemination for six months.

Question 2: If I'm a uterus owner, when should I consider an infertility workup?

If you want to get pregnant when you're forty or older, you may want to consider evaluation and treatment right away.

If you're between thirty-five and forty and you haven't gotten pregnant after six months of trying, or if you're under thirty-five and you haven't gotten pregnant after a year of trying, you should consider a workup.

Exception: If you have a condition that is known to put you at a higher risk for infertility (like PCOS or endometriosis), don't wait six months or a year. Ask your doctor if they think you should have a workup immediately.

Question 3: Why can't I get pregnant?

If you take a step back and look at the big picture, to get pregnant naturally, all these steps (also shown in figure 18) have to happen without a hitch:

- **The unfertilized egg's journey.** During a normal menstrual cycle, one of your ovaries releases a mature egg during a process called ovulation. In some cases, more than one egg can be released, which results in nonidentical twins or triplets. Interestingly, because of hormonal fluctuations that happen as a woman ages, women over thirty-five are more likely to release more than one egg a month. An egg can only survive for twenty-four hours in the fallopian tube. Eggs that are not fertilized either break down or flow out of the body (unnoticed) with vaginal secretions.

- **The sperm's journey.** Sperm must swim up through the cervix and the uterus, and then into the fallopian tube to fertilize the egg. Sperm can live in a woman's reproductive tract for five to seven days. It doesn't matter whether the sperm or the egg arrives first, but the egg and sperm must meet in the fallopian tube while both of them are still viable.

- **The fertilized egg's journey.** Once the egg and the sperm join, the fertilized egg has to travel down the fallopian tube into the uterus.
- **Implantation.** The fertilized egg implants (attaches) to the uterine wall and grows.

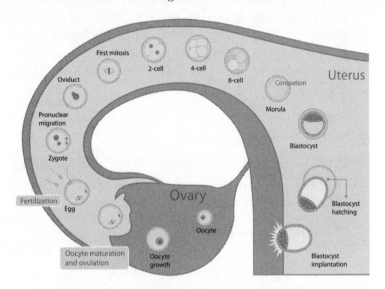

Figure 18. Summary of steps that occur during conception

Question 4: What are some common reasons for these steps to be disrupted?

- **Ovulation disorders.** Having a mature egg to fertilize is a nonnegotiable part of getting pregnant. There are lots of reasons women don't release an egg into the fallopian tube every month. For example, polycystic ovary syndrome (PCOS), which is a hormonal imbalance that frequently stops women from ovulating every month, is one of the most common causes of female infertility. For more information, see the Polycystic Ovarian Syndrome Spotlight (page 208).

Menopause is a natural part of life, not a disorder, but when a woman has ovaries that aren't producing eggs anymore, she is menopausal and she will not be able to get pregnant without in vitro fertilization (IVF). The average age of menopause is 51.4 years old. But during the years leading up to menopause, which are known as the menopause transition, a woman might not ovulate every month. The menopause transition usually lasts about seven years, but it can be as long as fifteen years.

- **Sperm issues.** Most people think of infertility as a "female problem." However, infertility can affect both women and men. In approximately 35 percent of couples with infertility, a male cause is identified in addition to a female cause, and in approximately 10 percent a male factor is the only cause. Men need to have a high concentration of fast sperm that are shaped correctly. These sperm have to be able to make it through the cervical mucus and travel through the uterus into the fallopian tubes. The sperm's journey to the egg is not easy.

- **Fallopian tube blockage.** Think of your fallopian tubes as the "street" between the uterus and ovaries. If the street is completely blocked for any reason, the egg and the sperm won't be able to find each other (figure 19). Or if it's partially blocked and they do manage to find each other, the fertilized egg might not be able to find its way back to the uterus. Some common reasons for blocked tubes include scar tissue that happens because of endometriosis, pelvic inflammatory disease from a past sexually transmitted disease (STD) — even if it happened decades ago (this is one of the many reasons teens need to know about safe sex) — or scar tissue from a past surgery in the pelvis or abdomen.

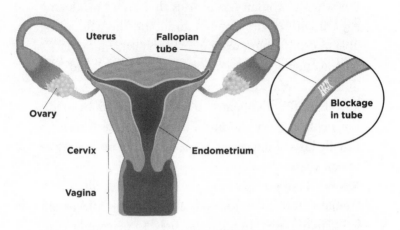

Figure 19. Blockage in fallopian tube that prevents the unfertilized egg, sperm, or fertilized egg from traveling freely

- **Implantation problems.** The fertilized egg could have a hard time implanting in the wall of the uterus because of issues like fibroids, polyps, or an unusually shaped uterus.

Question 5: If I need a workup, what would it involve?

Depending on your history and physical exam, your doctor will run tests to determine which issue(s) mentioned in question 4 is causing infertility. This list is not all-inclusive, but common go-to tests include the following:

Ovulation check. Here are four ways to check for ovulation:

- **Check your blood progesterone level.** Progesterone levels shoot up after ovulation. So progesterone levels are drawn approximately seven days after the date of suspected ovulation. If it is high, that usually means you ovulated that month. If your value is low, your doctor may recommend repeating the test in two or three days.

- **Use an at-home ovulation prediction kit.** These kits, available without a prescription, test your urine or saliva. However, they have a 5 to 10 percent chance of saying you are ovulating when you aren't, or aren't ovulating when you are.

- **Pay attention to what's happening with your menstrual cycle.** If you have a period about once a month, *and* you have premenstrual syndrome (PMS) symptoms like bloating or breast tenderness before your period starts, you are probably ovulating. Paying attention to the PMS symptoms is important because those symptoms are caused by the elevated level of progesterone that happens after ovulation. In addition to PMS symptoms, another clue that you are ovulating is if your vaginal discharge looks like raw egg whites. Typically, the cervix switches to this type of "sperm-friendly" discharge around the time of ovulation to help increase the chances of pregnancy.

- **Chart your basal body temperature.** Your basal body temperature is your temperature when you're fully at rest. It's taken right after you wake up and before you've had anything to eat or drink and before you've gotten out of bed and done any type of physical movement. One or two days after you ovulate, your body temperature will rise 0.5°F.

Egg health check. These labs, which may be done in conjunction with an ultrasound to look at your ovaries, give more information about the quality and quantity of eggs available for ovulation.

- **Anti-mullerian hormone (AMH).** AMH levels help determine how many potential eggs a woman has left for ovulation. If this level is very low, the probability of pregnancy is less likely and she may have a poor response to in vitro fertilization (IVF). This test can be done any time in the menstrual cycle.

- **Follicle stimulating hormone (FSH).** High levels of FSH implies that your pituitary gland needs to work really, really hard to stimulate the eggs in your ovaries. This could indicate a less than ideal quality or quantity of eggs in your ovaries. This lab is drawn on the third day of your period (where day one is the first day of full menstrual flow). Or, in some cases, instead of just checking a day-three FSH, your doctor will give you a medication called clomiphene citrate on days five through nine of your menstrual cycle and measure your FSH on menstrual cycle days three and ten. They may also check your estrogen level.

  If your doctor says your AMH is low or your FSH is high, I recommend that you ask to be referred to a reproductive endocrinology and infertility specialist, if you are not seeing one already. However, if your insurance doesn't cover the cost, it can be very expensive to see an infertility specialist.

Fallopian tube check. These are some of the commonly used tests that can determine if your "street" is blocked or damaged.

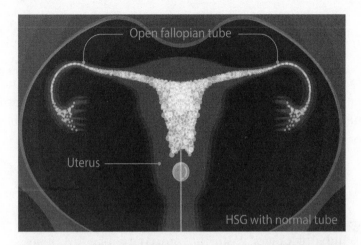

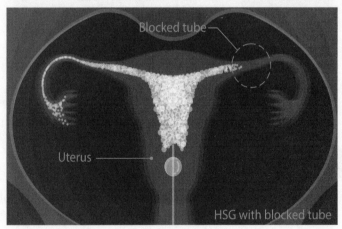

Figure 20. HSGs showing a uterus with two open fallopian tubes (*top*) and a uterus with one blocked fallopian tube (*bottom*)

- **Hysterosalpingogram** (HIS-te-ro-sal-PIN-go-gram; aka HSG). This is done by injecting dye into your uterus and then taking an X-ray to see if the dye flows through the uterus and spills out of your fallopian tubes (see figure 20). Ideally, you want both tubes to be open so that pregnancy is possible, regardless of which ovary releases the egg that month. But you can get pregnant with only one open fallopian tube. As an extra bonus, this test will also show problems inside the uterus, such as fibroids, polyps, or uterine malformations that you were born with.

- **Hysterosalpingo-contrast sonography** (aka Hy-CoSy) is an alternative. This uses an ultrasound to look at the uterus, tubes, and ovaries before and after injecting a combination of fluid with air.
- **Hysteroscopy.** A thin, lighted tube called a hysteroscope is used to determine if the tubes are open.
- **Chromopertubation** is another way to check for tube blockages. With this procedure, blue dye is injected into the uterus and then a camera is inserted into the abdomen during a surgery called a laparoscopy to see if the blue dye spills into your pelvis. If it does, that means the fallopian tube is open on that side. Laparoscopy also allows your doctor to look for and treat endometriosis, pelvic scar tissue, or other issues that may be causing or contributing to your infertility. Chromopertubation is performed in the operating room during the laparoscopy.

Note: In some situations, sometimes it looks like your tube is blocked on HSG or HyCoSy, but actually the tube is open but the injected material (e.g., the dye) couldn't get through because the tube had a spasm. Chromopertubation can be helpful in that situation.

Semen check. This ensures that the sperm are functioning properly and that there are enough of them to get the job done. The semen analysis should be collected after two to four days of abstinence, and you need to get it to the lab within one hour of collection.

Uterus check. There are lots of imaging options to assess your uterine cavity. These tests will make sure the fertilized egg has a comfy, cozy place to implant. Your practitioner will help you decide which test is best for you. They include:

- **Hysteroscopy.** A small, lighted camera is inserted into your uterus. If an abnormality is seen (e.g., a fibroid), it can be removed during this procedure.
- **Transvaginal ultrasound.** This procedure uses sound waves to create pictures of your uterus and ovaries.
- **Saline infusion sonohysterography (SIS).** Saline is injected into the uterus through the cervix to look at your uterine cavity during a transvaginal ultrasound.
- **Magnetic resonance imaging (MRI).** This uses a magnetic field and radio waves to create images of your internal organs and tissues.
- **HSG or HyCoSy.** See descriptions in fallopian tube check section above.

Depending on what your testing shows, your doctor might recommend one of these:

- **Laparoscopy.** This is a minimally invasive surgery that involves making a small incision beneath your navel. The doctor then inserts a small camera to look at your ovaries, uterus, and fallopian tubes. During a laparoscopy, endometriosis, scarring, fallopian tube irregularities, or problems with the uterus or ovaries can be seen and treated.
- **Genetic testing.** These tests would determine if any changes in your genes may be causing infertility or a greater chance to have a miscarriage.
- **General hormone check.** These labs are for checking other hormones such as prolactin, thyroid, or other reproductive hormones.

Sometimes, even after doing all these tests, the exact cause of infertility is never found. However, even if you don't find an exact cause, your doctor can still discuss treatment options with you to help you conceive faster than normal. And sometimes unexplained infertility corrects itself with time.

Question 6: What are the treatment options?

- **Dealing with ovulation disorders.** Oral or injected fertility medication may be used to help you ovulate. In general, your chance of getting pregnant is highest if you have sex one to two days before ovulation or on the day of ovulation.
- **Dealing with blocked tubes.** Surgery to unblock the fallopian tubes is an option. However, this surgery is not always recommended, since pregnancy chances are better with in vitro fertilization (IVF) than they would be if the tubes were surgically unblocked. If you choose IVF, your doctor might actually recommend having your tubes surgically removed or blocking the tubes close to the uterus because that may improve your chances of getting pregnant with IVF.
- **Dealing with sperm issues (or using donor sperm).** If sperm needs some help reaching the egg for any reason, intrauterine insemination (IUI) may be recommended. With IUI, a small catheter is used to place millions of healthy sperm inside the uterus around the time of ovulation. That puts them super close to the egg hanging out in the fallopian tube. Sometimes, this treatment is combined with fertility meds to help ovulation.
- **Dealing with uterine anatomy problems.** You may need surgery to correct the uterine anatomy problem(s). For instance, removing fibroids.
- **Dealing with any infertility issue discussed.** In vitro fertilization (IVF). No matter what the cause of

your infertility is, IVF may be helpful. After hormone injections, mature eggs are removed from a woman's ovaries and fertilized with sperm in a dish in the lab. After two to five days, the fertilized egg or eggs are put into your uterus. Hopefully, one of the fertilized eggs will attach to the wall of the uterus and grow into a pregnancy. IVF is currently the most aggressive tool we have to treat infertility. But since it's so expensive, and not all insurance plans cover it, not everyone has access to this option.

Make sure you ask your doctor about the risks and benefits of each treatment option. Also remember that an ob-gyn can start this workup and offer basic treatments, but if cost is not an issue you might want to think about seeing a reproductive endocrinologist and infertility specialist, especially if you're thirty-five or older or if you don't conceive after a few months of treatment from your ob-gyn.

DR. NITA'S NOTE
Don't Be "That Person"

I've seen "infertility bingo cards" floating around on social media. In the comments section of these posts, women dealing with infertility bond over the unhelpful things that well-meaning people say. If you know someone who's impacted by infertility, please don't say any of these things. I know your heart might be in the right place, but most women don't like hearing these types of comments or questions.

Infertility BINGO

B	I	N	G	O
Try (insert some random suggestion with no scientific basis).	If it's in God's plan, it'll happen.	I bet you're having fun trying!	You're lucky you don't have kids because (insert a reason that doesn't make you feel lucky).	(Insert some random person's name) got pregnant right after they adopted.
You shouldn't have waited so long to try.	Kids are overrated.	You're young. You have all the time in the world.	How long have you been trying?	Are you pregnant yet?
Just go on vacation.	I know how you feel.	My coworker's neighbor's niece tried for years, but now she's pregnant.	Maybe you're just too stressed. Try to relax.	What's meant to be will be.
You can have my kids.	Just do IVF.	Just adopt.	Do the doctors know why you can't get pregnant?	It will happen when you stop trying.
Why don't you just get a surrogate?	Try drinking more wine to loosen up.	At least it's not cancer.	Don't worry. It'll happen.	At least you already have a child.

Pregnancy Loss

The terminology for pregnancy loss can get confusing. In the United States, a miscarriage is usually defined as the loss of a baby before the twentieth week of pregnancy. A stillbirth is the loss of a baby at or after twenty weeks of pregnancy. The chapter introduction was about miscarriages worldwide, so the researchers used a different definition. But for the following questions, we will focus on miscarriages using the US definition.

Question 7: What causes a miscarriage?

Miscarriage is not your fault. About 60 percent of miscarriages happen because the fertilized egg has more or fewer chromosomes than the normal amount.[2] Therefore, the fetus doesn't develop as expected. These chromosome problems aren't typically due to problems inherited from parents. Instead, they frequently happen because of errors that occur by chance as the baby is developing. That's why most people usually go on to have healthy pregnancies after a miscarriage.

Eight out of ten miscarriages happen before the thirteenth week of pregnancy.[3]

Question 8: What's the likelihood of having another miscarriage?

Miscarriages are usually a one-time event. Only 2 percent of pregnant women experience two pregnancy losses in a row, and only about 1 percent have three consecutive pregnancy losses.[4] But remember that these are just average percentages. Age and lifestyle issues, such as smoking, have a big impact on individual risks.

Question 9: Will trying again too soon increase my chance of another miscarriage?

Delaying pregnancy does not decrease the risk of a repeat pregnancy loss. So whenever your doctor gives you the green light and you feel emotionally ready, go for it! For people who have had one miscarriage, doctors usually tell patients not to have sex or put anything in the vagina for two weeks to give the body time to heal and to prevent infection. For people who have had two or more miscarriages, the doctor might recommend waiting longer before trying to get pregnant again. They may want to draw labs to determine if they can find a treatable underlying cause that increases the risk of miscarriage.

Infertility and Miscarriages

Question 10: What can I do to increase my chances of getting pregnant if I have infertility or if I'm trying to get pregnant after having a miscarriage?[5]

Miscarriage

- If you're taking any medications, ask your doctor to review your meds and supplements list. Some medications and supplements are not safe during pregnancy.
- Avoid a body temperature of 100°F or more.
- Avoid environmental chemicals like pesticides.
- Limit caffeine intake to 200 mg a day or less.
- Avoid exposure to radiation.
- Avoid certain infections.

Infertility

- Do activities that will give you a sense of well-being, and try to avoid unnecessary stress. Having a sense of well-being and decreasing overall stress have been shown to increase the likelihood that IVF and intra-uterine insemination will be successful.
- If you have a low AMH level, ask your healthcare practitioner if you should consider taking an antioxidant. Antioxidants prevent the formation of free radicals in cells that lead to cellular damage and cell death. This may prevent aging of the egg and may promote more accurate chromosomal separation when cells divide. One option is Coenzyme Q_{10} (CoQ_{10}) 100 to 300 mg once or twice a day.

Note: Manufacturers of vitamin or herbal supplements are not required to have their product tested for an improvement or a correction of an infertility problem. Since supplements do not undergo rigorous testing, make sure you discuss this suggestion with your fertility doctor before proceeding.

Miscarriages and infertility

- Avoid tobacco, alcohol, and drugs.
- Maintain a healthy weight.
- Get medical issues like thyroid disease, diabetes, or high blood pressure under control.

Also, to prepare your body for pregnancy, take a prenatal vitamin containing folic acid, ideally starting at least three months before you get pregnant. Folic acid helps prevent neural tube defects, which are serious abnormalities of the fetal brain and spinal cord.

DR. NITA'S NOTE

Advocate for Your Health Like a Pro When Dealing with Infertility or Miscarriages

Here are some questions to ask your doctor:

Infertility

1. *Based on my history, what causes of infertility are you evaluating?* As your workup progresses, make sure you have a clear understanding of which causes have been ruled out and which are still being evaluated.

2. *Do I need to see a fertility specialist, or will you be able to help me?* Assuming you are not seeing a specialist already, even if you are not interested in IVF, you may want to consider a consultation with one, just to make sure you understand all the less-invasive treatment options.

3. *May I speak to someone in your billing department to get an estimate of how much the workup will cost?* If you are paying out of pocket, the individuals in the billing department (billers) may not be able to tell you exactly, but they might be able to give you a ballpark figure to help you plan accordingly. If your insurance company is involved, billers may ask you to call your insurance company to help determine how much you'll end up paying out-of-pocket. Tip: Some routine tests and imaging that are ordered for issues like heavy or painful periods are also needed for an infertility workup. Therefore, if you have abnormal uterine bleeding, for example, your insurance will probably cover the cost if your ob-gyn codes it as abnormal uterine bleeding instead of infertility. If your insurance

doesn't cover infertility, this tip may provide a little financial relief.

4. *Are there any programs that can help with the cost of medication?* There are lots of helpful programs, especially if you are doing IVF.

5. *Do I have any underlying medical conditions that need to be better controlled?* For example, if you know that you have diabetes or thyroid disease and you desire another pregnancy, ideally, you want to make sure they are under control before conceiving.

Miscarriage

1. *What is my blood type? Do I need a RhoGAM shot?* If you are Rh negative, you may need this shot to prevent the development of antibodies that could be harmful to a fetus in a future pregnancy.

2. *Do I have any underlying medical conditions that need to be better controlled?* For example, if you know that you have diabetes or thyroid disease and you desire another pregnancy, ideally, you want to make sure they are under control before conceiving.

3. (If you've had more than one miscarriage) *Do I need blood work to try to determine why I had another miscarriage?* Some practitioners will order labs after two miscarriages.

Infertility or Miscarriage

Let your doctor know if you would like to be referred to a therapist. About 20 percent of women who experience a miscarriage become symptomatic for anxiety or depression, and most of these women will have persistent symptoms for one to three years — these symptoms can even persist during and after a successful pregnancy.[6] And one study showed that out of two hundred couples that visited a fertility clinic, half of the women and 15 percent of the men said that infertility was the most upsetting experience of their lives.[7]

Also, joining online or in-person support groups can be incredibly beneficial. Infertility is hard. Miscarriages are hard. The emotional health of the birthing and nonbirthing parents is important. You don't have to do this alone.

Chapter 16

Transgender Health and Becoming a Respectful Ally

I interviewed several transgender people for this chapter. I was given permission to use names and other identifying information.

Meet Corinne Goodwin. She is a transgender woman — someone who was assigned male at birth but who identifies as female.

By the time she was three years old, she already felt like a girl. In fact, she was so sure that she was a girl that after she found out that her friend had "something different down there," she wondered how her parents had glued a penis onto her body. So she knew her truth before she learned her ABCs. But the people around her made it clear to young Corinne that they weren't on board with that truth.

She was teased mercilessly as a child, including by her grandfather, for being "girly." And when she was twelve years old, she was caught stealing women's clothing from a store. Her mother's response? "Instead of telling me that kleptomania is bad, she spent an entire evening telling me that I would be the cause of my father's death if he found out about my deviancy." Corinne was crushed. She didn't want to lose her family's love, so she decided to put their desires above her own, continuing to move through life as male.

When she was twenty-one, she fell in love and married a cisgender woman, and they eventually had a child. During their marriage, Corinne's wife did all she could to be supportive, including spending an average of one weekend a month visiting her mother out of town so that Corinne could have an extended period of time presenting as her true female self. But at the age of fifty, Corinne knew that wasn't enough. If she was ever going to be truly happy, she couldn't go on living as a man. So with the loving support of the woman she *has been married to for forty years and counting*, Corinne transitioned into a life that allowed her outside appearance to match what she knew herself to be inside. And she now lives as the woman she was born to be. Corinne has gone through a lot, but she's quick to point out that it *does* get better.

Today, at sixty-two years old, Corinne is comfortable in her own skin and works tirelessly as the executive director of the Eastern Pennsylvania Trans Equity Project / Lehigh Valley Renaissance to promote the changes she knows the transgender community deserves. She hopes that sharing her experiences will help educate and inspire transgender people who are struggling to live as their authentic selves.

Meet Micah Rodriguez, a transgender man — someone who was assigned female at birth but who identifies as male:

Like Corinne, Micah knew he was transgender at an early age, but when he overheard his mother say that RuPaul, drag queen extraordinaire, was "disgusting," he thought to himself, "I can never tell my mother that this is who I am because if she thinks that's disgusting, God knows what she's going to think of me." So instead of disappointing his mom and family, he decided, like so many others, to hide his truth from the world.

To cope with the pressure, stress, and disappointment of living a lie, he turned to drugs.

But then Micah got a serious wakeup call when one of his friends overdosed and died. That's when he knew that he had to change his life, and fast. He stopped using drugs and moved to a new city for a fresh start. Then, at the age of thirty-two, *began the process of transitioning.*

Today Micah is a forty-year-old man experiencing a level of happiness he never could have experienced as a woman. It took some time, but now he has a great relationship with his family, including his mother, who loves him for who he is.

Of course, every transgender person's journey is unique, and some transgender people face more challenges than others. Dr. Gene de Haan, a nonbinary, transmasculine ob-gyn who specializes primarily in gender-affirming surgical care, stresses the importance of community resilience and celebration, which is just as critical as understanding the struggles and experiences of marginalization. De Haan states, "I am proud to be trans, and grateful for our vibrant and diverse communities."

Healthcare for Trans People

Regarding healthcare for transgender individuals, these are Dr. de Hann's tips:

- Find a practitioner who is gender affirming and well educated in gender-affirming care.
- Be mindful that the transgender community has a long history of needing to educate practitioners on the medical needs of transgender people. Trans patients have historically been the experts on their own care, and this is still the case in many parts of the country and world.

- Many gender-affirming practitioners see patients virtually, so if someone does not feel supported — or worse, if they are experiencing overt transphobia — they should find a different practitioner.
- There are many clinics in different parts of the country, like Callen-Lorde, Lyon-Martin, and Fenway Health, that have a long history of serving the LGBTQIA+ (lesbian, gay, bisexual, transgender, queer/questioning, intersex, asexual, and other) community. Depending on where people live, these clinics may be a great resource.
- There are services that people can research online. It's also a great idea to talk to friends and community if they have access to them.

Tips for Being a Respectful Ally

In an effort to learn more about ways to support the LGBTQIA+ community, I asked Corinne, Micah, Dr. de Haan, and the mother of a transgender child how readers can become respectful allies. These are their top suggestions.

1. Understand the basics

- Sex assigned at birth is based on your genital anatomy at birth — typically, male or female (unless you are intersex, that is, born with anatomy that doesn't seem to fit the typical definitions of female or male). Sex assigned at birth is usually documented on your birth certificate.
- Gender has nothing to do with a person's genital anatomy. It's based on how a person *feels* on the inside, on the spectrum of masculinity, femininity, or androgyny

(androgyny means neither specifically masculine nor feminine).

- When someone's *sex assigned at birth* matches their *gender*, they are *cisgender*.
- When someone's sex assigned at birth doesn't match their gender, they may identify as transgender, nonbinary, or gender nonconforming.

2. Use the right pronouns

Regardless of what a transgender person decides about hormones or surgery, and no matter how they might look to you (facial hair, no facial hair, high-pitched voice, deep voice, breast tissue, no breast tissue), call them by the pronouns that represent their identity. If you aren't sure what pronouns they prefer, there's a simple solution: ask them. For example, "Hi, my name is Nita, and my pronouns are she/her. What about you?"

A few of the common pronouns include (you'll notice that some of these are gender neutral because some people don't identify as a specific gender):

- She/her. *She is a really nice person. I really like her.*
- He/him. *He is a really nice person. I really like him.*
- They/them. *They are a really nice person. I really like them.*
- Ze/hir (*Ze* is usually pronounced with a long *e. Hir* is usually pronounced like the word *here.*) *Ze is a very nice person. I really like hir.*
- Ze/zir (*Zir* is usually pronounced with a long *e* as in *here.*) *Ze is a really nice person. I really like zir.*
- Some people prefer to go by their name, or if you're having a hard time remembering their pronouns, you're always safe using their name. *(Insert name) is a really nice person. I really like (insert name).*

How big a deal are pronouns? They are a huge deal! Every person I interviewed talked about the emotional pain of being misgendered. Corinne equates being called the wrong pronoun day after day with feeling like "death by a thousand paper cuts."

3. Don't ask about surgeries

"So ... have you had *the* operation yet?" the lady asked.

People ask Corinne Goodwin, a transgender woman, this kind of stuff all the time. So she wasn't surprised that the woman she had met just a few minutes earlier felt comfortable asking her this question as they sat down at the table at a dinner party.

But instead of getting upset, Corinne decided to use the situation as a teachable moment. Maintaining her composure, she turned to the woman (who obviously believed that asking strangers for the deets on their nether regions was socially acceptable small talk), and said, "I'm happy to answer that question, but can I ask you a question first? When was the last time a stranger asked you about your vagina?"

Then Corinne patiently waited for a response. But she was met with deafening silence, which probably meant that the answer to her question was, "Since I'm a cisgender, heterosexual woman, strangers don't ask me personal questions about my genitals."

4. Avoid insensitive questions and comments

Here are some things you should never say:

- Don't ask them their "real" name, and never call them by their deadname. Their deadname reminds them of a time when they were being forced to take on an identity that didn't fit them. If he introduces himself as Greg, his name is Greg. Period.

- Don't ask, "Are you sure you're not just super gay?" This question is hella rude. Plus, sexual orientation, which reflects who a person is attracted to, is a totally different topic. A transgender person might be attracted to the same sex, the opposite sex, or both sexes.
- Don't say, "Wow, you look just like a real man/woman." That isn't a compliment. They *are* a real man or woman.
- Don't tell transgender jokes. They are hurtful.
- Don't out someone as trans to a third party without permission. Don't say, "By the way, he's transgender." They are capable of sharing that information if they want to. You can, of course, tell someone the proper pronouns to use, but if you do, offer your own pronouns as well.
- Don't ask them how they have sex. Because it's none of your business.
- Don't ask them, "Are you going to change your mind?" They don't need you to question them. Instead, opt for these three key phrases that Corinne says every transgender person wants to hear when they come out to you: (1) "Thank you for telling me"; (2) "This won't change our relationship"; and (3) "Please let me know how I can be an ally."

5. Stand up for trans people being disrespected

If you see a transgender person being treated unfairly, here's how you can help.

Corinne introduced me to the STOP method for when

you see someone treating a transgender person disrespectfully (whether or not the person who is being rude is aware of it): *S*ay what's wrong, *T*ell them why, *O*ffer a new way of doing it, *P*ractice. So if you hear someone misgendering a trans person, stop them and say, "You're using the wrong pronouns, and that makes me feel uncomfortable." Then say, "Her pronouns are she/her. If you practice, you'll be able to remember, or just use her name."

6. Support transgender kids

One of the mothers I interviewed wanted to give parents of transgender kids some advice. "My son was always very masculine as a toddler, but I didn't think much about it. It just never occurred to me that my son was trans. I didn't even know the word. I still went through typical stages of grief, including denial."

In retrospect, she now realizes that if a child comes out as trans, you can bet they've felt that way for a long time. You may feel blindsided, but they aren't. Her best advice is to:

1. believe your child when they tell you who they are;
2. send them to transgender-affirming places so they can meet other trans kids;
3. stick up for them out in the world; and
4. affirm that you love them no matter what.

I also like Corinne's suggestion to remember that the situation isn't about you or what your neighbors might think. It's about your child's physical and emotional health. So she states that you should research the local resources, and get support for both of you.

Transgender Health and Becoming a Respectful Ally: The Wrap-Up

While I don't have enough experience with the resources listed below to personally endorse them, some of the transgender individuals who were interviewed for this book stated that these resources are well-respected and helpful. And many more resources are available to help you find community, information, and physical/emotional healthcare. Don't forget to search for services in your specific area. Remember that help is available — and that you deserve it.

- American College of Obstetricians and Gynecologists: https://www.acog.org
- *Comprehensive Care of the Transgender Patient*, 1st edition, by Cecile A. Ferrando, MD, MPH
- Endocrine Society: https://www.endocrine.org/advocacy /position-statements/transgender-health
- The Gay and Lesbian Medical Association (GLMA), including a database to help you search for healthcare practitioners: https://www.glma.org
- GLAAD's list of transgender resources: https://www.glaad.org/transgender/resources
- GLSEN provides resources that support LGBTQIA+ youth in our schools: https://www.glsen.org/
- National Center for Transgender Equality: https://transequality.org
- National LGBTQIA+ Health Education Center: https://www.lgbtqiahealtheducation.org/resources /in/transgender-health
- Pediatric Endocrine Society: https://pedsendo.org/?s=transgender
- PFLAG provides resources to LGBTQIA+ individuals, their families, and allies: https://pflag.org

- Planned Parenthood, which provides transgender services: https://plannedparenthood.org
- Trans Lifeline (hotline for information and support): 877-565-8860, https://translifeline.org
- The Trevor Project (crisis and suicide prevention): 866-488-7386, https://thetrevorproject.org
- UCSF Center of Excellence for Transgender Health: https://prevention.ucsf.edu/transhealth
- The World Professional Association for Transgender Health: https://www.wpath.org/soc8

Before I Say Goodbye

In *The War of Art*, Steven Pressfield explains that most of us have two lives: the life we live and the life we are capable of living.

Be honest with yourself. When it comes to your sexual and physical health, are you truly living your best life? If you aren't, today is a perfect day to start changing your narrative! As you use the information written in this book, here's a checklist to get you started:

- ❏ Be willing to take the steps you need to take to create the types of sexual experiences you truly desire.
- ❏ Put in the work to stay physically healthy.
- ❏ Actively search for practitioners who see you, respect you, and listen to you.
- ❏ Vow to never stop advocating for your health.
- ❏ Always remember that you *deserve* to be the healthiest, happiest version of yourself.

Cheers to better sex, better health, and a better you,

Dr. Nita ♥

Acknowledgments

First and foremost, I'd like to thank my parents for their love, support, and guidance. I'd also like to give a big shout-out to my sisters, Tonya, Carm, and Lenski. Thanks for being an endless reservoir of comic relief when I need a work break. (And for occasionally forcing me to take work breaks that I need but don't desire.) I wouldn't trade our shenanigans for anything in the world.

Of course, this book would not be what it is without the incredible support and talent from the team at New World Library. To my editorial director, Georgia Hughes, and my managing editor, Kristen Cashman, whew! Words cannot express how appreciative I am for your patience. Thank you for your guidance, and thank you for giving me a perfect balance of direction, time, space, and creative freedom to carefully craft each chapter. I definitely owe you dinner and a cocktail (or two)! Tracy Cunningham, thanks for the amazing illustrations and the fabulous cover. Tona Pearce Myers, thanks for bringing it all together. And to Monique Muhlenkamp and everyone else who contributed their time and expertise, thank you!

To my agent, Greg A. Ray, thank you for believing in the vision for this book from day one. I will be forever grateful for your support (and your inspirational emojis).

To everyone at *The Doctors* TV show, thanks for giving me a platform that allowed me to merge two of my passions: medicine and entertainment.

And a huge thank-you to everyone who agreed to be interviewed or read portions of the book and provided feedback. I cannot stress how much I appreciate your time and suggestions! Thank you, thank you, thank you to:

Dr. Linda Bradley, Dr. Patti Britton, Dr. Yolanda Cavalier, Dr. Shannon Chavez, Dr. Gene de Haan, Dr. Rosalyn Dischiavo, Dr. Alyssa Dweck, Dr. Kristi Funk, Dr. Paria Hassouri, Dr. Hal Leland, Dr. Mary Jane Minkin, Dr. Patti Leeke Mwesigwa, Dr. Stephen Nakajima, Dr. Leah Nakamura, Dr. Rachel Needle, Dr. Ina Park, Dr. Lynn Parker, Dr. Jennifer Perkins, Dr. Botros Rizk, Dr. Saloni Sharma, Dr. Aaron Spitz, Dr. Lauren Streicher, Dr. Shontell Thomas, Dr. Michelle Uaje, Ashley Amey, Jovanka Ciares, Nicole Collins, Misti Johnson Cowherd, Bailey Gaddis, Corinne Goodwin, Sandra Mesics, Fatima Muse, Lauren Phillips, Micah Rodriguez, Anthony Schaeffer, and Darrelyn Smith.

And to everyone who has given me the honor of being their doctor, thank you.

Appendix A

CDC Screening Recommendations and Considerations for STDs

The table below summarizes the screening recommendations from the Centers for Disease Control and Prevention.[1]

Chlamydia	
Women	• Sexually active women under 25 years of age • Sexually active women 25 years of age and older if at increased risk* • Retest approximately 3 months after treatment • Rectal chlamydial testing can be considered in females based on reported sexual behaviors and exposure, through shared clinical decision between the patient and the provider.

Chlamydia *(continued)*	
Pregnant women	• All pregnant women under 25 years of age • Pregnant women 25 years of age and older if at increased risk* • Retest during the third trimester for women under 25 years of age or at risk • Pregnant women with chlamydial infection should have a test of cure 4 weeks after treatment and be retested within 3 months
Men who have sex with women	• There is insufficient evidence for screening among heterosexual men who are at low risk for infection; however, screening young men can be considered in high-prevalence clinical settings (adolescent clinics, correctional facilities, STI/sexual health clinics)
Men who have sex with men (MSM)	• At least annually for sexually active MSM at sites of contact (urethra, rectum) regardless of condom use • Every 3 to 6 months if at increased risk (i.e., MSM on PrEP, with HIV infection, or if they or their sex partners have multiple partners)
Transgender and gender-diverse persons	• Screening recommendations should be adapted based on anatomy, (i.e., annual, routine screening for chlamydia in cisgender women younger than 25 years old should be extended to all transgender men and gender diverse people with a cervix. If over 25 years old, persons with a cervix should be screened if at increased risk.) • Consider screening at the rectal site based on reported sexual behaviors and exposure

Chlamydia (*continued*)	
Persons with HIV	• For sexually active individuals, screen at the first HIV evaluation, and at least annually thereafter. • More frequent screening might be appropriate depending on individual risk behaviors and the local epidemiology

* Per U.S. Preventive Services Task Force, women 25 years or older are at increased risk for chlamydial and gonococcal infections if they have a new partner, more than one sex partner, a sex partner with concurrent partners, or a sex partner who has an STI; practice inconsistent condom use when not in a mutually monogamous relationship; have a previous or coexisting STI; have a history of exchanging sex for money or drugs; or have a history of incarceration.

Gonorrhea	
Women	• Sexually active women under 25 years of age • Sexually active women 25 years of age and older if at increased risk* • Retest 3 months after treatment • Pharyngeal and rectal gonorrhea screening can be considered in females based on reported sexual behaviors and exposure, through shared clinical decision between the patient and the provider.
Pregnant women	• All pregnant women under 25 years of age, and those 25 and older if at increased risk* • Retest during the 3rd trimester for women under 25 years of age or at risk • Pregnant women with gonorrhea should be retested within 3 months
Men who have sex with women	• There is insufficient evidence for screening among heterosexual men who are at low risk for infection

Gonorrhea *(continued)*	
Men who have sex with men (MSM)	• At least annually for sexually active MSM at sites of contact (urethra, rectum, pharynx) regardless of condom use • Every 3 to 6 months if at increased risk
Transgender and gender-diverse persons	• Screening recommendations should be adapted based on anatomy (i.e., annual, routine screening for gonorrhea in cisgender women younger than 25 years old should be extended to all transgender men and gender diverse people with a cervix. If over 25 years old, screen if at increased risk.) • Consider screening at the pharyngeal and rectal site based on reported sexual behaviors and exposure
Persons with HIV	• For sexually active individuals, screen at first HIV evaluation, and at least annually thereafter • More frequent screening might be appropriate depending on individual risk behaviors and the local epidemiology

* Per U.S. Preventive Services Task Force, women 25 years or older are at increased risk for chlamydial and gonococcal infections if they have a new partner, more than one sex partner, a sex partner with concurrent partners, or a sex partner who has an STI; practice inconsistent condom use when not in a mutually monogamous relationship; have a previous or coexisting STI; have a history of exchanging sex for money or drugs; or have a history of incarceration.

Hepatitis B	
Women	• Women at increased risk (having had more than one sex partner in the previous 6 months, evaluation or treatment for an STI, past or current injection-drug use, and an HBsAg-positive sex partner)

Hepatitis B *(continued)*	
Pregnant women	• Test for HBsAg at the first prenatal visit of each pregnancy regardless of prior testing; retest at delivery if at high risk
Men who have sex with women	• Men at increased risk (i.e., by sexual or percutaneous exposure)
Men who have sex with men (MSM)	• All MSM should be tested for HBsAg, anti-HBc, and anti-HBs
Persons with HIV	• Test for HBsAg, anti-HBc, and anti-HBs

Hepatitis C	
Women	• All adults over age 18 years should be screened for hepatitis C except in settings where the hepatitis C infection (HCV) positivity is less than 0.1 percent
Pregnant women	• Pregnant women should be screened for hepatitis C except in settings where the hepatitis C infection (HCV) positivity is less than 0.1 percent
Men who have sex with women	• All adults over age 18 years should be screened for hepatitis C except in settings where the hepatitis C infection (HCV) positivity is less than 0.1 percent
Men who have sex with men (MSM)	• All adults over age 18 years should be screened for hepatitis C except in settings where the hepatitis C infection (HCV) positivity is less than 0.1 percent
Persons with HIV	• Serologic testing at initial evaluation • Annual HCV testing in MSM with HIV infection

Herpes[†]	
Women	• Type-specific HSV serologic testing can be considered for women presenting for an STI evaluation (especially for women with multiple sex partners)
Pregnant women	• Routine HSV-2 serologic screening among asymptomatic pregnant women is not recommended. However, type-specific serologic tests might be useful for identifying pregnant women at risk for HSV infection and guiding counseling regarding the risk for acquiring genital herpes during pregnancy
Men who have sex with women	• Type-specific HSV serologic testing can be considered for men presenting for an STI evaluation (especially for men with multiple sex partners)
Men who have sex with men (MSM)	• Type-specific serologic tests can be considered if infection status is unknown in MSM with previously undiagnosed genital tract infection
Persons with HIV	• Type-specific HSV serologic testing should be considered for persons presenting for an STI evaluation (especially for those persons with multiple sex partners)

†   Type-specific HSV-2 serologic assays for diagnosing HSV-2 are useful in the following scenarios: recurrent or atypical genital symptoms or lesions with a negative HSV PCR or culture result, clinical diagnosis of genital herpes without laboratory confirmation, and a patient's partner has genital herpes. HSV-2 serologic screening among the general population is not recommended. Patients who are at higher risk for infection (e.g., those presenting for an STI evaluation, especially for persons with 10 or more lifetime sex partners, and persons with HIV infection) might need to be assessed for a history of genital herpes symptoms, followed by type-specific HSV serologic assays to diagnose genital herpes for those with genital symptoms.

HIV	
Women	• All women aged 13 to 64 years, unless the patient declines[‡] • All women who seek evaluation and treatment for STIs
Pregnant women	• All pregnant women should be screened at first prenatal visit, unless the patient declines • Retest in the third trimester if at high risk (people who use drugs, have STIs during pregnancy, have multiple sex partners during pregnancy, have a new sex partner during pregnancy, live in areas with high HIV prevalence, or have partners with HIV) • Rapid testing should be performed at delivery if not previously screened during pregnancy
Men who have sex with women	• All men aged 13 to 64 years, unless the patient declines[‡] • All men who seek evaluation and treatment for STIs
Men who have sex with men (MSM)	• At least annually for sexually active MSM if HIV status is unknown or negative and the patient or their sex partner(s) have had more than one sex partner since most recent HIV test • Consider the benefits of offering more frequent HIV screening (e.g., every 3 to 6 months) to MSM at increased risk for acquiring HIV infection
Transgender and gender-diverse persons	• HIV screening should be discussed and offered to all transgender persons. Frequency of repeat screenings should be based on level of risk.

[‡] The United States Preventative Services Task Force (USPSTF) recommends screening in adults and adolescents ages 15 to 65.

HPV, Cervical Cancer, Anal Cancer[§]	
Women	• Women 21 to 29 years of age every 3 years with cytology • Women 30 to 65 years of age every 3 years with cytology, or every 5 years with a combination of cytology and HPV testing
Pregnant women	• Pregnant women should be screened at the same intervals as nonpregnant women.
Men who have sex with men (MSM)	• Digital anorectal rectal exam • Data is insufficient to recommend routine anal cancer screening with anal cytology
Transgender and gender-diverse people	• Screening for people with a cervix should follow current screening guidelines for cervical cancer
Persons with HIV	• Providers should defer to existing *Guidelines for the Prevention and Treatment of Opportunistic Infections in Adults and Adolescents with HIV* for guidance on cervical cancer screening and management of results in persons with HIV

§   Data are insufficient to recommend routine anal cancer screening with anal cytology among populations at risk for anal cancer. Certain clinical centers perform anal cytology to screen for anal cancer among populations at high risk (e.g., persons with HIV infection, MSM, and those having receptive anal intercourse), followed by high-resolution anoscopy (HRA) for those with abnormal cytologic results (e.g., ASC-US, LSIL, or HSIL).

Syphilis	
Women	• Screen asymptomatic women at increased risk (history of incarceration or transactional sex work, geography, race/ethnicity) for syphilis infection.
Pregnant women	• All pregnant women at the first prenatal visit • Retest at 28 weeks gestation and at delivery if at high risk (lives in a community with high syphilis morbidity or is at risk for syphilis acquisition during pregnancy [drug misuse, STIs during pregnancy, multiple partners, a new partner, partner with STIs])
Men who have sex with women	• Screen asymptomatic adults at increased risk (history of incarceration or transactional sex work, geography, race/ethnicity, and being a male younger than 29 years) for syphilis infection
Men who have sex with men (MSM)	• At least annually for sexually active MSM • Every 3 to 6 months if at increased risk • Screen asymptomatic adults at increased risk (history of incarceration or transactional sex work, geography, race/ethnicity, and being a male younger than 29 years) for syphilis infection
Transgender and gender-diverse people	• Consider screening at least annually based on reported sexual behaviors and exposure
Persons with HIV	• For sexually active individuals, screen at first HIV evaluation, and at least annually thereafter • More frequent screening might be appropriate depending on individual risk behaviors and the local epidemiology

Trichomoniasis	
Women	• Consider screening for women receiving care in high-prevalence settings (e.g., STI clinics and correctional facilities) and for asymptomatic women at high risk for infection (e.g., women with multiple sex partners, transactional sex, drug misuse, or a history of STI or incarceration)
Persons with HIV	• Recommended for sexually active women at entry to care and at least annually thereafter

Appendix B

Summary Chart of U.S. Medical Eligibility Criteria for Contraceptive Use

This detailed chart from the CDC indicates how all the common birth control methods interact with a huge variety of medical conditions.[1] How to use this chart:

1. Find the birth control method you're interested in using at the top. (I = initiation; C = continuation)
   - Cu-IUD = Copper intrauterine device
   - LNG-IUD = Any progestin-containing intrauterine device (brand names: Mirena, Liletta, Kyleena, Skyla)
   - Implant = Arm implant (brand name: Nexplanon)
   - DMPA = Birth control shot (brand name: Depo-Provera)
   - POP = Progestin-only birth control pill
   - CHC = Combined hormonal contraception (birth control pills with estrogen and progestin, the vaginal birth control ring, the birth control patch)
2. Find your medical condition in the two left-hand columns.

3. Look at where your birth control method and your condition intersect. Here's what each number means:
    ○   1 = You're good to go! The method can be used safely. ("No restriction.")
    ○   2 = Some risk is involved, but it's still safe. ("Advantages generally outweigh theoretical or proven risks.")
    ○   3 = You should pick another method. ("Theoretical or proven risks usually outweigh the advantages.")
    ○   4= Abort! Do not use this method. ("Unacceptable health risk.")

Examples:

Breast disease → Undiagnosed mass → Copper IUD = 1 = You're good to go!

Breast disease → Undiagnosed mass → LNG-IUD = 2 = Some risk is involved, but it's still safe.

Summary Chart of U.S. Medical Eligibility Criteria for Contraceptive Use

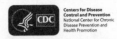

Centers for Disease Control and Prevention
National Center for Chronic Disease Prevention and Health Promotion

Condition	Sub-Condition	Cu-IUD I	Cu-IUD C	LNG-IUD I	LNG-IUD C	Implant I	Implant C	DMPA I	DMPA C	POP I	POP C	CHC I	CHC C
Age		Menarche to <20 yrs:2 / ≥20 yrs:1		Menarche to <20 yrs:2 / ≥20 yrs:1 / >45=1		Menarche to <18 yrs:1 / 18-45 yrs:1 / >45 yrs:1		Menarche to <18 yrs:2 / 18-45 yrs:1 / >45 yrs:2		Menarche to <18 yrs:1 / 18-45 yrs:1 / >45 yrs:1		Menarche to <40 yrs:1 / ≥40 yrs:2	
Anatomical abnormalities	a) Distorted uterine cavity	4	4	4	4								
	b) Other abnormalities	2	2	2	2								
Anemias	a) Thalassemia	2	2	1	1	1	1	1	1	1	1	1	1
	b) Sickle cell disease‡	2	2	1	1	1	1	1	1	1	1	2	2
	c) Iron-deficiency anemia	2	2	1	1	1	1	1	1	1	1	1	1
Benign ovarian tumors	(including cysts)	1	1	1	1	1	1	1	1	1	1	1	1
Breast disease	a) Undiagnosed mass	1	1	2	2	2*	2*	2*	2*	2*	2*	2*	2*
	b) Benign breast disease	1	1	1	1	1	1	1	1	1	1	1	1
	c) Family history of cancer	1	1	1	1	1	1	1	1	1	1	1	1
	d) Breast cancer‡												
	i) Current	1	1	4	4	4	4	4	4	4	4	4	4
	ii) Past and no evidence of current disease for 5 years	1	1	3	3	3	3	3	3	3	3	3	3
Breastfeeding	a) <21 days postpartum					2*	2*	2*	2*	2*	2*	4*	4*
	b) 21 to <30 days postpartum												
	i) With other risk factors for VTE					2*	2*	2*	2*	2*	2*	3*	3*
	ii) Without other risk factors for VTE					2*	2*	2*	2*	2*	2*	3*	3*
	c) 30-42 days postpartum												
	i) With other risk factors for VTE					1*	1*	1*	1*	1*	1*	3*	3*
	ii) Without other risk factors for VTE					1*	1*	1*	1*	1*	1*	2*	2*
	d) >42 days postpartum					1*	1*	1*	1*	1*	1*	2*	2*
Cervical cancer	Awaiting treatment	4	2	4	2	2	2	2	2	1	1	2	2
Cervical ectropion		1	1	1	1	1	1	1	1	1	1	1	1
Cervical intraepithelial neoplasia		1	1	2	2	2	2	2	2	1	1	2	2
Cirrhosis	a) Mild (compensated)	1	1	1	1	1	1	1	1	1	1	1	1
	b) Severe‡ (decompensated)	1	1	3	3	3	3	3	3	3	3	4	4
Cystic fibrosis‡		1*	1*	1*	1*	1*	1*	2*	2*	1*	1*	1*	1*
Deep venous thrombosis (DVT)/Pulmonary embolism (PE)	a) History of DVT/PE, not receiving anticoagulant therapy												
	i) Higher risk for recurrent DVT/PE	1	1	2	2	2	2	2	2	2	2	4	4
	ii) Lower risk for recurrent DVT/PE	1	1	2	2	2	2	2	2	2	2	3	3
	b) Acute DVT/PE	2	2	2	2	2	2	2	2	2	2	4	4
	c) DVT/PE and established anticoagulant therapy for at least 3 months												
	i) Higher risk for recurrent DVT/PE	2	2	2	2	2	2	2	2	2	2	4*	4*
	ii) Lower risk for recurrent DVT/PE	2	2	2	2	2	2	2	2	2	2	3*	3*
	d) Family history (first-degree relatives)	1	1	1	1	1	1	1	1	1	1	2	2
	e) Major surgery												
	i) With prolonged immobilization	1	1	2	2	2	2	2	2	2	2	4	4
	ii) Without prolonged immobilization	1	1	1	1	1	1	1	1	1	1	2	2
	f) Minor surgery without immobilization	1	1	1	1	1	1	1	1	1	1	1	1
Depressive disorders		1*	1*	1*	1*	1*	1*	1*	1*	1*	1*	1*	1*

Key:

1 No restriction (method can be used)	3 Theoretical or proven risks usually outweigh the advantages
2 Advantages generally outweigh theoretical or proven risks	4 Unacceptable health risk (method not to be used)

Summary Chart of U.S. Medical Eligibility Criteria for Contraceptive Use

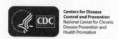

Centers for Disease Control and Prevention
National Center for Chronic Disease Prevention and Health Promotion

Condition	Sub-Condition	Cu-IUD I	Cu-IUD C	LNG-IUD I	LNG-IUD C	Implant I	Implant C	DMPA I	DMPA C	POP I	POP C	CHC I	CHC C
Diabetes	a) History of gestational disease	1		1		1		1		1		1	
	b) Nonvascular disease												
	i) Non-insulin dependent	1		2		2		2		2		2	
	ii) Insulin dependent	1		2		2		2		2		2	
	c) Nephropathy/retinopathy/neuropathy[‡]	1		2		2		3		2		3/4*	
	d) Other vascular disease or diabetes of >20 years' duration[‡]	1		2		2		3		2		3/4*	
Dysmenorrhea	Severe	2		1		1		1		1		1	
Endometrial cancer[‡]		4	2	4	2	1		1		1		1	
Endometrial hyperplasia		1		1		1		1		1		1	
Endometriosis		2		1		1		1		1		1	
Epilepsy[‡]	(see also Drug Interactions)	1		1		1*		1*		1*		1*	
Gallbladder disease	a) Symptomatic												
	i) Treated by cholecystectomy	1		2		2		2		2		2	
	ii) Medically treated	1		2		2		2		2		3	
	iii) Current	1		2		2		2		2		3	
	b) Asymptomatic	1		2		2		2		2		2	
Gestational trophoblastic disease[‡]	a) Suspected GTD (immediate postevacuation)												
	i) Uterine size first trimester	1*		1*		1*		1*		1*		1*	
	ii) Uterine size second trimester	2*		2*		1*		1*		1*		1*	
	b) Confirmed GTD												
	i) Undetectable/non-pregnant ß-hCG levels	1*	1*	1*	1*	1*		1*		1*		1*	
	ii) Decreasing ß-hCG levels	2*	1*	2*	1*	1*		1*		1*		1*	
	iii) Persistently elevated ß-hCG levels or malignant disease, with no evidence or suspicion of intrauterine disease	2*	1*	2*	1*	1*		1*		1*		1*	
	iv) Persistently elevated ß-hCG levels or malignant disease, with evidence or suspicion of intrauterine disease	4*	2*	4*	2*	1*		1*		1*		1*	
Headaches	a) Nonmigraine (mild or severe)	1		1		1		1		1		1*	
	b) Migraine												
	i) Without aura (includes menstrual migraine)	1		1		1		1		1		2*	
	ii) With aura	1		1		1		1		1		4*	
History of bariatric surgery[‡]	a) Restrictive procedures	1		1		1		1		1		1	
	b) Malabsorptive procedures	1		1		1		1		3		COCs: 3 P/R: 1	
History of cholestasis	a) Pregnancy related	1		1		1		1		1		2	
	b) Past COC related	1		2		2		2		2		3	
History of high blood pressure during pregnancy		1		1		1		1		1		2	
History of Pelvic surgery		1		1		1		1		1		1	
HIV	a) High risk for HIV	1*	1*	1*	1*	1		1		1		1	
	b) HIV infection					1*		1*		1*		1*	
	i) Clinically well receiving ARV therapy	1	1	1	1	If on treatment, see Drug Interactions							
	ii) Not clinically well or not receiving ARV therapy[‡]	2	1	2	1	If on treatment, see Drug Interactions							

Abbreviations: ARV = antiretroviral; C=continuation of contraceptive method; CHC=combined hormonal contraception (pill, patch, and, ring); COC=combined oral contraceptive; Cu-IUD=copper-containing intrauterine device; DMPA = depot medroxyprogesterone acetate; I=initiation of contraceptive method; LNG-IUD=levonorgestrel-releasing intrauterine device; NA=not applicable; POP=progestin-only pill; P/R=patch/ring; SSRI=selective serotonin reuptake inhibitor; ‡ Condition that exposes a woman to increased risk as a result of pregnancy. *Please see the complete guidance for a clarification to this classification: https://www.cdc.gov/reproductivehealth/contraception/contraception_guidance.htm

Summary Chart of U.S. Medical Eligibility Criteria for Contraceptive Use

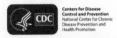

Centers for Disease
Control and Prevention
National Center for Chronic
Disease Prevention and
Health Promotion

Condition	Sub-Condition	Cu-IUD I	Cu-IUD C	LNG-IUD I	LNG-IUD C	Implant I	Implant C	DMPA I	DMPA C	POP I	POP C	CHC I	CHC C
Hypertension	a) Adequately controlled hypertension	1*		1*		1*		2*		1*		3*	
	b) Elevated blood pressure levels (*properly taken measurements*)												
	i) Systolic 140-159 or diastolic 90-99	1*		1*		1*		2*		1*		3*	
	ii) Systolic ≥160 or diastolic ≥100‡	1*		2*		2*		3*		2*		4*	
	c) Vascular disease	1*		2*		2*		3*		2*		4*	
Inflammatory bowel disease	(*Ulcerative colitis, Crohn's disease*)	1		1		1		2		2		2/3*	
Ischemic heart disease‡	Current and history of	1		2	3	2	3	3		2	3	4	
Known thrombogenic mutations‡		1*		2*		2*		2*		2*		4*	
Liver tumors	a) Benign												
	i) Focal nodular hyperplasia	1		2		2		2		2		2	
	ii) Hepatocellular adenoma‡	1		3		3		3		3		4	
	b) Malignant‡ (hepatoma)	1		3		3		3		3		4	
Malaria		1		1		1		1		1		1	
Multiple risk factors for atherosclerotic cardiovascular disease	(e.g., older age, smoking, diabetes, hypertension, low HDL, high LDL, or high triglyceride levels)	1		2		2*		3*		2*		3/4*	
Multiple sclerosis	a) With prolonged immobility	1		1		1		2		1		3	
	b) Without prolonged immobility	1		1		1		2		1		1	
Obesity	a) Body mass index (BMI) ≥30 kg/m²	1		1		1		1		1		2	
	b) Menarche to <18 years and BMI ≥ 30 kg/m²	1		1		1		2		1		2	
Ovarian cancer‡		1		1		1		1		1		1	
Parity	a) Nulliparous	2		2		1		1		1		1	
	b) Parous	1		1		1		1		1		1	
Past ectopic pregnancy		1		1		1		1		2		1	
Pelvic inflammatory disease	a) Past												
	i) With subsequent pregnancy	1	1	1	1	1		1		1		1	
	ii) Without subsequent pregnancy	2	2	2	2	1		1		1		1	
	b) Current	4	2*	4	2*	1		1		1		1	
Peripartum cardiomyopathy‡	a) Normal or mildly impaired cardiac function												
	i) <6 months	2		2		1		1		1		4	
	ii) ≥6 months	2		2		1		1		1		3	
	b) Moderately or severely impaired cardiac function	2		2		2		2		2		4	
Postabortion	a) First trimester	1*		1*		1*		1*		1*		1*	
	b) Second trimester	2*		2*		1*		1*		1*		1*	
	c) Immediate postseptic abortion	4		4		1*		1*		1*		1*	
Postpartum (*nonbreastfeeding women*)	a) <21 days							1		1		4	
	b) 21 days to 42 days												
	i) With other risk factors for VTE							1		1		3*	
	ii) Without other risk factors for VTE							1		1		2	
	c) >42 days							1		1		1	
Postpartum (*in breastfeeding or non-breastfeeding women, including cesarean delivery*)	a) <10 minutes after delivery of the placenta												
	i) Breastfeeding	1*		2*									
	ii) Nonbreastfeeding	1*		1*									
	b) 10 minutes after delivery of the placenta to <4 weeks	2*		2*									
	c) ≥4 weeks	1*		1*									
	d) Postpartum sepsis	4		4									

Summary Chart of U.S. Medical Eligibility Criteria for Contraceptive Use

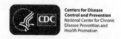

Centers for Disease Control and Prevention
National Center for Chronic Disease Prevention and Health Promotion

Condition	Sub-Condition	Cu-IUD		LNG-IUD		Implant		DMPA		POP		CHC	
		I	C	I	C	I	C	I	C	I	C	I	C
Pregnancy		4*		4*		NA*		NA*		NA*		NA*	
Rheumatoid arthritis	a) On immunosuppressive therapy	2	1	2	1	1		2/3*		1		2	
	b) Not on immunosuppressive therapy	1		1		1		2		1		2	
Schistosomiasis	a) Uncomplicated	1		1		1		1		1		1	
	b) Fibrosis of the liver‡	1		1		1		1		1		1	
Sexually transmitted diseases (STDs)	a) Current purulent cervicitis or chlamydial infection or gonococcal infection	4	2*	4	2*	1		1		1		1	
	b) Vaginitis (including trichomonas vaginalis and bacterial vaginosis)	2	2	2	2	1		1		1		1	
	c) Other factors relating to STDs	2*	2	2*	2	1		1		1		1	
Smoking	a) Age <35	1		1		1		1		1		2	
	b) Age ≥35, <15 cigarettes/day	1		1		1		1		1		3	
	c) Age ≥35, ≥15 cigarettes/day	1		1		1		1		1		4	
Solid organ transplantation‡	a) Complicated	3	2	3	2	2		2		2		4	
	b) Uncomplicated	2		2		2		2		2		2*	
Stroke‡	History of cerebrovascular accident	1		2		2	3	3		2	3	4	
Superficial venous disorders	a) Varicose veins	1		1		1		1		1		1	
	b) Superficial venous thrombosis (acute or history)	1		1		1		1		1		3*	
Systemic lupus erythematosus‡	a) Positive (or unknown) antiphospholipid antibodies	1*	1*	3*		3*		3*	3*	3*		4*	
	b) Severe thrombocytopenia	3*	2*	2*		2*		3*	2*	2*		2*	
	c) Immunosuppressive therapy	2*	1*	2*		2*		2*	2*	2*		2*	
	d) None of the above	1*	1*	2*		2*		2*	2*	2*		2*	
Thyroid disorders	Simple goiter/ hyperthyroid/hypothyroid	1		1		1		1		1		1	
Tuberculosis‡ (see also Drug Interactions)	a) Nonpelvic	1	1	1	1	1*		1*		1*		1*	
	b) Pelvic	4	3	4	3	1*		1*		1*		1*	
Unexplained vaginal bleeding	(suspicious for serious condition) before evaluation	4*	2*	4*	2*	3*		3*		2*		2*	
Uterine fibroids		2		2		1		1		1		1	
Valvular heart disease	a) Uncomplicated	1		1		1		1		1		2	
	b) Complicated‡	1		1		1		1		1		4	
Vaginal bleeding patterns	a) Irregular pattern without heavy bleeding	1		1	1	2		2		2		1	
	b) Heavy or prolonged bleeding	2*		1*	2*	2*		2*		2*		1*	
Viral hepatitis	a) Acute or flare	1		1		1		1		1		3/4*	2
	b) Carrier/Chronic	1		1		1		1		1		1	1
Drug Interactions													
Antiretrovirals used for prevention (PrEP) or treatment of HIV	Fosamprenavir (FPV)	1/2*	1*	1/2*	1*	2*		2*		2*		3*	
	All other ARVs are 1 or 2 for all methods.												
Anticonvulsant therapy	a) Certain anticonvulsants (phenytoin, carbamazepine, barbiturates, primidone, topiramate, oxcarbazepine)	1		1		2*		1*		3*		3*	
	b) Lamotrigine	1		1		1		1		1		3*	
Antimicrobial therapy	a) Broad spectrum antibiotics	1		1		1		1		1		1	
	b) Antifungals	1		1		1		1		1		1	
	c) Antiparasitics	1		1		1		1		1		1	
	d) Rifampin or rifabutin therapy	1		1		2*		1*		3*		3*	
SSRIs		1		1		1		1		1		1	
St. John's wort		1		1		2		1		2		2	

Appendix C

Bladder Training Instructions

As mentioned in chapter 12, bladder training can help incontinence. Here's how to do it:

- Empty your bladder as soon as you wake up in the morning.
- During the day, go to the bathroom at the specific time intervals that you and your healthcare practitioner have discussed. To start off, this may mean peeing every hour during the day. At night, only go to the bathroom if you wake up and find it necessary. If you urinate a lot at night, avoid drinking fluids three to four hours before going to bed.
- When you go to the bathroom at your scheduled times, attempt to urinate whether or not you feel like you need to, even if you have just experienced urinary incontinence.
- If you feel a strong urge to urinate before your scheduled time, don't run to the bathroom. Instead:
  - Stop what you are doing (freeze).

- ○ Do three Kegels (squeeze).
- ○ Take some deep breaths as you try to distract yourself.
- ○ Once you feel in control, walk slowly to the bathroom and urinate.
- Once you can go two days without urinary incontinence, increase the time between scheduled toilet trips by fifteen minutes. Once you go two days without having incontinence on your new schedule, increase it by another fifteen minutes. Keep doing this until you can go four hours between toilet trips (that is normal). It may take several weeks to reach your four-hour goal. Hang in there!

Reputable Resources

The following organizations provide a wealth of easy-to-understand information on women's health.

- American College of Obstetricians and Gynecologists: https://www.acog.org
- Cleveland Clinic: https://my.clevelandclinic.org
- Johns Hopkins: https://www.hopkinsmedicine.org
- Mayo Clinic: https://www.mayoclinic.org
- Office on Women's Health: https://www.womens health.gov

Notes

Chapter 1. Misconceptions about Sex

1. David A. Frederick et al., "Differences in Orgasm Frequency Among Gay, Lesbian, Bisexual, and Heterosexual Men and Women in a U.S. National Sample," *Archives of Sexual Behavior* 47 (2018): 273–88, https://doi.org/10.1007/s10508-017-0939-z.

Chapter 2. Anatomy

1. Shere Hite, *The Hite Report: A Nationwide Study of Female Sexuality* (New York: Macmillan, 1976).
2. Rachel N. Pauls, "Anatomy of the Clitoris and the Female Sexual Response," *Clinical Anatomy* 28, no. 3 (2015): 376–84, doi:10.1002/ca.22524.
3. "Female Genital Anatomy," Boston University School of Medicine, accessed July 28, 2021, https://www.bumc.bu.edu/sexualmedicine/physicianinformation/female-genital-anatomy.
4. Kim Wallen and Elizabeth A. Lloyd, "Female Sexual Arousal: Genital Anatomy and Orgasm in Intercourse," *Hormones and Behavior* 59, no. 5 (2011): 780–92, https://doi.org/10.1016/j.yhbeh.2010.12.004.
5. Ihab Younis, Menhaabdel Fattah, and Marwa Maamon, "Female Hot Spots: Extragenital Erogenous Zones," *Human Andrology* 6, no. 1 (March 2016): 20–26, doi:10.1097/01.XHA.0000481142.54302.08.
6. Zlatko Pastor, "Female Ejaculation Orgasm vs. Coital Incontinence:

A Systematic Review," *Journal of Sexual Medicine* 10, no. 7 (July 2013): 1682–91, doi: 10.1111/jsm.12166.

7. Samuel Salama et al., "Nature and Origin of 'Squirting' in Female Sexuality," *Journal of Sexual Medicine* 12, no. 3 (March 2015): 661–66, doi: 10.1111/jsm.12799.

Chapter 3. Desire, Arousal, and Orgasms

1. Rosemary Basson, "The Female Sexual Response: A Different Model," *Journal of Sex & Marital Therapy* 26, no. 1 (2000): 51–65, doi: 10.1080/009262300278641.

2. A. Dubinskaya et al., "Local Genital Arousal: Mechanisms for Vaginal Lubrication," *Current Sexual Health Reports* 13 (June 2021): 45–53, https://doi.org/10.1007/s11930-021-00305-8.

3. Emily Nagoski, *Come As You Are: The Surprising New Science That Will Transform Your Sex Life* (New York: Simon & Schuster, 2015), 42–67.

4. J. R. Berman, "Physiology of Female Sexual Function and Dysfunction," *International Journal of Impotence Research* 17 (2005): S44–S51, https://doi.org/10.1038/sj.ijir.3901428.

5. Hepeng Zhang et al., "miR-137 Affects Vaginal Lubrication in Female Sexual Dysfunction by Targeting Aquaporin-2," *Sexual Medicine* 6, no. 4 (December 2018): 339–47, doi: 10.1016/j.esxm.2018.09.002.

6. Hannah Frith, *Orgasmic Bodies: The Orgasm in Contemporary Western Culture* (London: Palgrave Macmillan, 2015), https://doi.org/10.1057/9781137304377_2.

7. James G. Pfaus et al., "The Whole Versus the Sum of Some of the Parts: Toward Resolving the Apparent Controversy of Clitoral Versus Vaginal Orgasms," *Socioaffective Neuroscience and Psychology* 6, no. 32578 (October 2016), https://doi.org/10.3402/snp.v6.32578.

Chapter 4. Diagnosing and Treating Sexual Dysfunction

1. Jan L. Shifren, Brigitta U. Monz, Patricia A. Russo, Anthony Segreti, and Catherine B. Johannes, "Sexual Problems and Distress in United States Women: Prevalence and Correlates," *Obstetrics & Gynecology* 112, no. 5 (November 2008): 970–78, doi: 10.1097/AOG.0b013e318 1898cdb.

2. Dr. Jessica O'Reilly, *The Doctors*, "The Sexologist Answers Your Questions about Sex and Foreplay!," October 9, 2020, https://www.thedoctorstv.com/videos/the-sexologist-answers-your-questions-about-sex-and-foreplay.

3. Christian C. Joyal, Amélie Cossette, and Vanessa Lapierre, "What Exactly Is an Unusual Sexual Fantasy?," *Journal of Sexual Medicine* 12, no. 2 (2015): 328–40.

4. Erick Janssen and John Bancroft, "The Dual-Control Model: The Role of Sexual Inhibition & Excitation in Sexual Arousal and Behavior," in *The Psychophysiology of Sex*, ed. Erik Janssen (Bloomington: Indiana University Press, 2006), 197–222; Bancroft et al., "The Dual Control Model: Current Status and Future Directions," *Journal of Sex Research* 46, no. 2–3 (2009): 121–42, doi: 10.1080/00224490902747222.

5. "Elective Female Genital Cosmetic Surgery," American College of Obstetricians and Gynecologists, Committee Opinion no. 795 (January 2020), https://www.acog.org/clinical/clinical-guidance/committee-opinion/articles/2020/01/elective-female-genital-cosmetic-surgery.

6. "One of Dr. Maya Angelou's Most Important Life Lessons," The Oprah Winfrey Show, aired June 18, 1997, https://www.oprah.com/own-oprah show/one-of-dr-maya-angelous-most-important-lessons_1, accessed July 11, 2022.

7. These two lists are adapted from the United Nations, "What Is Domestic Abuse?," accessed July 11, 2022, https://www.un.org/en/coronavirus/what-is-domestic-abuse.

8. "Devastatingly Pervasive: 1 in 3 Women Globally Experience Violence," World Health Organization, March 9, 2021, https://www.who.int/news/item/09-03-2021-devastatingly-pervasive-1-in-3-women-globally-experience-violence.

Chapter 5. Sexually Transmitted Infections and Diseases

1. "Chlamydia – CDC Fact Sheet (Detailed)," Centers for Disease Control and Prevention, last reviewed April 12, 2022, https://www.cdc.gov/std/chlamydia/stdfact-chlamydia-detailed.htm.

2. "What You Need to Know about the Links Between HIV and STDs," New York State Department of Health, accessed August 4, 2021, https://www.google.com/url?q=https://www.health.ny.gov/diseases/aids/consumers/hiv_basics/stds_hiv.htm&sa=D&source=editors&ust=1628103308114000&usg=AOvVaw3xyBcTYj3bTxYY99MAPZzX.

3. "Frequently Asked Questions (FAQs) about Condoms," New York State Department of Health, accessed August 4, 2021, https://www.health.ny.gov/diseases/aids/consumers/condoms/faqs.htm.

4. "What Type of Lube Is Best for Anal Sex?," San Francisco City Clinic, accessed August 4, 2021, https://www.sfcityclinic.org/faq/what-type-lube-best-anal-sex.

5. Katherine Hsu, "Treatment of Chlamydia Trachomatis Infection," *Up-ToDate*, last updated July 2, 2021, https://www.uptodate.com/contents/treatment-of-chlamydia-trachomatis-infection?search=chlamydia&source=search_result&selectedTitle=1~150&usage_type=default&display_rank=1#H343038.

6. Arlene C. Seña and Myron S. Cohen, "Treatment of Uncomplicated Neisseria Gonorrhoeae Infections," *UpToDate*, last updated January 27, 2022, https://www.uptodate.com/contents/treatment-of-uncomplicated-neisseria-gonorrhoeae-infections?search=gonorrhea&source=search_result&selectedTitle=1~150&usage_type=default&display_rank=1#H4144073. See also "Gonorrhea — CDC Face Sheet," Centers for Disease Control and Prevention, last reviewed April 12, 2022, https://www.cdc.gov/std/gonorrhea/stdfact-gonorrhea.htm.

7. "Syphilis Treatment and Care," Centers for Disease Control and Prevention, last reviewed January 3, 2022, https://www.cdc.gov/std/syphilis/treatment.htm.

8. "Trichomoniasis," Centers for Disease Control and Prevention, accessed August 4, 2021, https://www.cdc.gov/std/trichomonas/the-facts/trichomoniasis_bro_508.pdf.

9. "Pre-Exposure Prophylaxis (PrEP)," Centers for Disease Control and Prevention, last reviewed August 6, 2021, https://www.cdc.gov/hiv/risk/prep/index.html.

10. "Genital Herpes," Johns-Hopkins Medicine, accessed June 13, 2022, https://www.hopkinsmedicine.org/health/conditions-and-diseases/herpes-hsv1-and-hsv2/genital-herpes.

11. Geraldine McQuillan, Deanna Kruszon-Moran, Elaine W. Flagg, and Ryne Paulose-Ram, "Prevalence of Herpes Simplex Virus Type 1 and Type 2 in Persons Aged 14–49: United States, 2015–2016," NCHS Data Brief No. 304, February 2018, https://www.cdc.gov/nchs/products/databriefs/db304.htm#:~:text=The%20prevalence%20of%20HSV%2D1,and%2040%E2%80%9349%2C%20respectively.

12. Theresa Hoke et al., "Female Condoms," *UpToDate*, last updated October 7, 2021, https://www.uptodate.com/contents/female-condoms?search=internal%20condom&source=search_result&selectedTitle=1~150&usage_type=default&display_rank=1#H3.

13. "Female Condom," American Pregnancy Association, accessed August 4, 2021, https://americanpregnancy.org/unplanned-pregnancy/birth-control-pills-patches-and-devices/female-condom/.

14. "Basic Information about HPV and Cancer," Centers for Disease Control and Prevention, last reviewed December 13, 2021, https://www.cdc.gov/cancer/hpv/basic_info/index.htm.

15.   "Chlamydia Trachomatis: Symptoms & Causes," Mayo Clinic, accessed
      August 4, 2021, https://www.mayoclinic.org/diseases-conditions
      /chlamydia/symptoms-causes/syc-20355349.

16.   "Genital Herpes: Symptoms & Causes," Mayo Clinic, accessed August
      4, 2021, https://www.mayoclinic.org/diseases-conditions/genital-herpes
      /symptoms-causes/syc-20356161.

17.   "HPV Infection: Symptoms & Causes," Mayo Clinic, accessed August 4,
      2021, https://www.mayoclinic.org/diseases-conditions/hpv-infection
      /diagnosis-treatment/drc-20351602.

18.   "Syphilis: Symptoms & Causes," Mayo Clinic, accessed August 4, 2021,
      https://www.mayoclinic.org/diseases-conditions/syphilis
      /symptoms-causes/syc-20351756.

19.   "Syphilis: Symptoms & Causes," Mayo Clinic.

20.   "Retesting after Treatment to Detect Repeat Infections," Centers for
      Disease Control and Prevention, Sexually Transmitted Infection Treat-
      ment Guidelines, 2021, last reviewed July 22, 2021, https://www.cdc
      .gov/std/treatment-guidelines/clinical-retesting.htm.

21.   "How to Tell Someone That You Have an STD or STI," Cleveland
      Clinic, July 21, 2021, https://health.clevelandclinic.org/h-how-to-tell
      -your-partner-you-have-an-std/.

Chapter 6. Tips for Finding a Doctor You Actually Like

1.   Brad N. Greenwood et al., "Physician-Patient Racial Concordance and
     Disparities in Birthing Mortality for Newborns," *Proceedings of the National
     Academy of Sciences* 117, no. 35 (September 2020): 21, 194–21, 200;
     https://doi.org/10.1073/pnas.1913405117.

2.   "Why Are Black Women at Such High Risk of Dying from Pregnancy
     Complications?," *American Heart Association News*, February 20, 2019,
     https://www.heart.org/en/news/2019/02/20/why-are-black-women
     -at-such-high-risk-of-dying-from-pregnancy-complications.

3.   "Severe Maternal Morbidity: New York City, 2008–2012," New York
     City Department of Health and Mental Hygiene, Bureau of Maternal,
     Infant and Reproductive Health, accessed July 1, 2021, https://www1
     .nyc.gov/assets/doh/downloads/pdf/data/maternal-morbidity-report
     -08-12.pdf.

4.   Colleen Walsh, "COVID-19 Targets Communities of Color," *Harvard
     Gazette*, April 14, 2020, https://news.harvard.edu/gazette/story
     /2020/04/health-care-disparities-in-the-age-of-coronavirus/.

5.   Janice Sabin et al., "Physicians' Implicit and Explicit Attitudes about

Race by MD Race, Ethnicity, and Gender," *Journal of Health Care for the Poor and Underserved* 20, no. 3 (2009): 896–913, doi: 10.1353/hpu.0.0185.

6. James Madara, "Speaking Out Against Structural Racism at JAMA and Across Health Care," AMA, March 10, 2021, https://www.ama-assn .org/about/leadership/speaking-out-against-structural-racism-jama -and-across-health-care; "Ending Structural Racism," National Institutes of Health, accessed September 30, 2021, https://www.nih .gov/ending-structural-racism; Zinzi D. Bailey et al., "How Structural Racism Works — Racist Policies as a Root Cause of U.S. Racial Health Inequities," *New England Journal of Medicine* 384, no. 8 (2021): 768–73, doi:10.1056/NEJMms2025396; Bailey et al., "Structural Racism and Health Inequities in the USA: Evidence and Interventions," *Lancet* 389, no. 10077 (2017): 1453–63, doi: 10.1016/S0140-6736(17)30569-X.

7. Darshali A. Vyas et al., "Hidden in Plain Sight: Reconsidering the Use of Race Correction in Clinical Algorithms," *New England Journal of Medicine* 83, no. 9 (2020): 874–82, doi: 10.1056/NEJMms2004740.

Chapter 7. PMS and PMDD

1. Saskia Verkaik, Astrid M. Kamperman, Roos van Westrhenen, and Peter F.J. Schulte, "The Treatment of Premenstrual Syndrome with Preparations of Vitex Agnus Castus: A Systematic Review and Meta-analysis," *American Journal of Obstetrics and Gynecology* 217, no. 2 (2017): 150–66, doi: 10.1016/j.ajog.2017.02.028, https://www.sciencedirect .com/science/article/pii/S0002937817303198.

2. Giulia Dante and Fabio Facchinetti, "Herbal Treatments for Alleviating Premenstrual Symptoms: A Systematic Review," *Journal of Psychosomatic Obstetrics and Gynaecology* 32, no. 1 (2011): 42–51, doi: 10.3109/0167482X.2010.538102.

3. Mohamed F. M. Mitwally, Lynda Gotlieb, and Robert F. Casper, "Prevention of Bone Loss and Hypoestrogenic Symptoms by Estrogen and Interrupted Progestogen Add-Back in Long-Term GnRH-Agonist Down-Regulated Patients with Endometriosis and Premenstrual Syndrome," *Menopause* 9, no. 4 (2002): 236–41, doi: 10.1097/00042192 -200207000-00004; Mohamed Bedaiwy and Robert F. Casper, "Treatment with Leuprolide Acetate and Hormonal Add-Back for up to 10 Years in Stage IV Endometriosis Patients with Chronic Pelvic Pain," *Fertility and Sterility* 86, no. 1 (2006): 220–22, doi: 10.1016/j.fertnstert .2005.12.030.

Chapter 8. Period Pain

1. Roger P. Smith and Andrew M. Kaunitz, "Dysmenorrhea in Adult Females: Clinical Features and Diagnosis, *UpToDate*, last updated February 18, 2022, https://www.uptodate.com/contents/dysmenorrhea-in-adult-females-clinical-features-and-diagnosis?search=secondary%20dysmenorrhea&source=search_result&selectedTitle=1~150&usage_type=default&display_rank=1.

2. Amir H. Pakpour, "Depression, Anxiety, Stress, and Dysmenorrhea: A Protocol for a Systematic Review," *Systematic Reviews* 9, no. 1 (2020): article 65, https://doi.org/10.1186/s13643-020-01319-4.

Chapter 9: Periods That Are Heavy, Irregular, or Missing in Action

1. Charles J Glueck et al., "Pregnancy Outcomes among Women with Polycystic Ovary Syndrome Treated with Metformin," *Human Reproduction* 17, no. 11 (2002): 2858–64. doi: 10.1093/humrep/17.11.2858.

Chapter 10: Birth Control Cheat Sheet

1. James Trussell, "Contraceptive Failure in the United States," *Contraception* 83, no. 5 (May 2011): 397, doi: 10.1016/j.contraception.2011.01.021; Aparna Sundaram et al., "Contraceptive Failure in the United States: Estimates from the 2006–2010 National Survey of Family Growth," *Perspectives on Sexual and Reproductive Health* 49, no. 1 (2017): 7.

2. Tanja Baltus, James Brown, Sujana Molakatalla, and Supuni Kapurubandara, "Spontaneous Pregnancy after Total Bilateral Salpingectomy: A Systematic Review of Literature," *Journal of Minimally Invasive Gynecology* 29, no. 1 (September 2021), doi: 10.1016/j.jmig.2021.09.713.

3. "Depo-Provera: Prescribing Information," US FDA, accessed July 5, 2022, https://www.accessdata.fda.gov/drugsatfda_docs/label/2010/020246s036lbl.pdf.

4. "Committee Opinion: Depot Medroxyprogesterone Acetate and Bone Effects," American College of Obstetricians and Gynecologists, June 2014, https://www.acog.org/clinical/clinical-guidance/committee-opinion/articles/2014/06/depot-medroxyprogesterone-acetate-and-bone-effects.

5. "Emergency Contraception," Faculty of Sexual and Reproductive Healthcare of the Royal College of Obstetricians and Gynaecologists

(FSRH), last updated December 2020, https://www.fsrh.org/standards
-and-guidance/fsrh-guidelines-and-statements/emergency-contraception.

6.   "Oral Contraceptives and Cancer Risk," National Cancer Institute, last
      reviewed February 22, 2018, https://w ww.cancer.gov/about-cancer/
      causes-prevention/risk/hormones/oral-contraceptives-fact-sheet.

Chapter 11. Cancer Screening Guidelines

1.   "Breast Cancer Risk Factors You Cannot Change," American Cancer
      Society, accessed October 23, 2021, https://www.cancer.org/cancer
      /breast-cancer/risk-and-prevention/breast-cancer-risk-factors-you
      -cannot-change.html.

2.   "Screening for Breast Cancer: U.S. Preventive Services Task Force
      Recommendation Statement," *Annals of Internal Medicine* 151, no. 10
      (November 2009): 716, https://www.acpjournals.org/doi/10.7326/0003
      -4819-151-10-200911; Jan Peter Kösters and Peter C. Gøtzsche, "Reg-
      ular Self-Examination or Clinical Examination for Early Detection of
      Breast Cancer," *Cochrane Database of Systematic Reviews* 2003, no. 2 (2003):
      CD003373, https://doi.org/10.1002/14651858.CD003373; David B.
      Thomas et al., "Randomized Trial of Breast Self-Examination in
      Shanghai: Final Results," *Journal of the National Cancer Institute* 94, no. 19
      (2002): 1445–57, https://doi.org/10.1093/jnci/94.19.1445; Joshua J.
      Fenton et al., "Screening Clinical Breast Examination: How Often Does
      It Miss Lethal Breast Cancer?" *Journal of the National Cancer Institute Mono-
      graphs* 2005, no. 35 (2005): 67–71, https://doi.org/10.1093
      /jncimonographs/lgi040.

3.   Ralph J. Coates, "Patterns and Predictors of the Breast Cancer Detec-
      tion Methods in Women under Forty-Five Years of Age (United States),"
      Cancer Causes and Control 12 (2001): 431–42, https://www.semantic
      scholar.org/paper/Patterns-and-predictors-of-the-breast-cancer-in-45
      -Coates-Uhler/79e02352dc6f1a1f60731c85577995e45b0bf0b1; Laura
      M. Newcomer et al., "Detection Method and Breast Carcinoma Histol-
      ogy," *Cancer* 95, no. 3 (2002): 470–77, https://acsjournals.onlinelibrary
      .wiley.com/doi/full/10.1002/cncr.10695.

4.   "What Breast Cancer Can Look and Feel Like," Know Your Lemons
      Foundation, accessed July 5, 2022, https://knowyourlemons.org.

5.   "Breast Cancer Screening Guidelines for Women," Centers for Disease
      Control and Prevention, accessed October 20, 2021, https://www.cdc
      .gov/cancer/breast/pdf/breast-cancer-screening-guidelines-508.pdf.

6. Kevin C. Oeffinger et al., "Breast Cancer Screening for Women at Average Risk: 2015 Guideline Update from the American Cancer Society," *JAMA* 314, no. 15 (2015): 1599–614, doi: 10.1001/jama.2015.12783.

7. "Ovarian Cancer Risk Factors," American Cancer Society, last revised January 26, 2021, https://www.cancer.org/cancer/ovarian-cancer/causes-risks-prevention/risk-factors.html.

8. Michael J. Hall, "Lynch Syndrome (Hereditary Nonpolyposis Colorectal Cancer): Cancer Screening and Management," *UpToDate*, last updated February 22, 2022, https://www.uptodate.com/contents/lynch-syndrome-hereditary-nonpolyposis-colorectal-cancer-cancer-screening-and-management?search=lynch%20syndrome%20screening&source=search_result&selectedTitle=2~150&usage_type=default&display_rank=2#H1010647575.

Chapter 12: Urinary Incontinence

1. Carrie Carls, "The Prevalence of Stress Urinary Incontinence in High School and College-Age Female Athletes in the Midwest: Implications for Education and Prevention," *Urologic Nursing* 27, no. 1 (2007): 21–24, 39.

2. Rebecca G. Rogers and Tola B. Fashokun, "Pelvic Organ Prolapse in Women: Epidemiology, Risk Factors, Clinical Manifestations, and Management," *UpToDate*, last updated March 3, 2022, https://www.uptodate.com/contents/pelvic-organ-prolapse-in-women-epidemiology-risk-factors-clinical-manifestations-and-management?search=pelvic%20organ%20prolapse%20in%20women&source=search_result&selectedTitle=1~116&usage_type=default&display_rank=1.

Chapter 13: Caring for Your Vulva and Vagina

1. "Bacterial Vaginosis — CDC Fact Sheet," Centers for Disease Control and Prevention, last reviewed January 5, 2022, https://www.cdc.gov/std/bv/stdfact-bacterial-vaginosis.htm.

2. Liselotte Hardy et al., "Bacterial Biofilms in the Vagina," *Research in Microbiology* 168, no. 9–10 (2017): 865–74, doi: 10.1016/j.resmic.2017.02.001; Hyun-Sul Jung et al., "Etiology of Bacterial Vaginosis and Polymicrobial Biofilm Formation, *Critical Reviews in Microbiology* 43, no. 6 (2017): 651–67, doi: 10.1080/1040841X.2017.1291579.

3. Jennifer M. Fettweis et al., "Differences in Vaginal Microbiome in African American Women versus Women of European Ancestry," *Microbiology (Reading)* 160, pt. 10 (2014): 2272–82, doi: 10.1099/mic.0.081034-0.

4. Sophia Yen et al., "Bacterial Vaginosis in Sexually Experienced and Non-Sexually Experienced Young Women Entering the Military," *Obstetrics and Gynecology* 102, no. 5, pt. 1 (2003): 927–33, doi: 10.1016/s0029-7844(03)00858-5; Katherine A. Fethers et al., "Early Sexual Experiences and Risk Factors for Bacterial Vaginosis," *Journal of Infectious Diseases* 200, no. 11 (2009): 1662–70, doi: 10.1086/648092.

5. Jenifer E. Allsworth and Jeffrey F. Peipert, "Prevalence of Bacterial Vaginosis: 2001–2004 National Health and Nutrition Examination Survey Data," *Obstetrics and Gynecology* 109, no. 1 (January 2007): 114–20, doi: 10.1097/01.aog.0000247627.84791.91.

Chapter 14: When Your Hormones Go Off a Cliff

1. Barbara Kantrowitz and Pat Wingert, *The Menopause Book* (New York: Workman, 2017).

2. "Dealing with the Symptoms of Menopause," Harvard Medical School, *Harvard Health Publishing*, March 17, 2017, https://www.health.harvard.edu/womens-health/dealing-with-the-symptoms-of-menopause; "Menopause Transition: What's Normal?," Mayo Clinic, March 12, 2015, accessed January 7, 2022, https://www.mayoclinichealthsystem.org/hometown-health/speaking-of-health/menopause-transition; "Symptoms: Menopause," National Health Service, last reviewed August 29, 2021, https://www.nhs.uk/conditions/menopause/symptoms; Mark D. Grant et al., "Menopausal Symptoms: Comparative Effectiveness of Therapies," Agency for Healthcare Research and Quality (US), *Comparative Effectiveness Reviews*, no. 147 (March 2015), https://www.ncbi.nlm.nih.gov/books/NBK285446.

3. Richard Santen, Charles L. Loprinzi, and Robert F. Casper, "Menopausal Hot Flashes," *UpToDate*, last updated April 27, 2020, https://www.uptodate.com/contents/menopausal-hot-flashes?search=menopause%20transition&source=search_result&selectedTitle=7~150&usage_type=default&display_rank=7#H1.

4. Eleanor Mann et al., "Cognitive Behavioural Treatment for Women Who Have Menopausal Symptoms after Breast Cancer Treatment (MENOS 1): A Randomised Controlled Trial," *The Lancet: Oncology* 13, no. 3 (2012): 309–18, doi: 10.1016/S1470-2045(11)70364-3.

5. Kantrowitz and Wingert, *The Menopause Book*, 455.

6. Kantrowitz and Wingert, *The Menopause Book*, 455.

7. "Committee Opinion: Compounded Bioidentical Menopausal Hormone Therapy," American College of Obstetrics and Gynecologists Clinical, August 2012, https://www.acog.org/clinical/clinical-guidance /committee-opinion/articles/2012/08/compounded-bioidentical -menopausal-hormone-therapy.

Chapter 15: Miscarriages and Infertility

1. Siobhan Quenby et al., "Miscarriage Matters: The Epidemiological, Physical, Psychological, and Economic Costs of Early Pregnancy Loss," *Lancet* 397, no. 10285 (2021): 1658–67, doi: 10.1016/S0140-6736(21)00682-6.

2. "Repeated Miscarriages FAQs: What Is the Most Common Cause of Miscarriage?," American College of Obstetricians and Gynecologists," last reviewed November 2020, https://www.acog.org/womens-health /faqs/repeated-miscarriages.

3. L. Regan and R. Rai, "Epidemiology and the Medical Causes of Miscarriage," *Bailliere's Best Practice & Research, Clinical Obstetrics & Gynaecology* 14, no. 5 (2000): 839–54. doi: 10.1053/beog.2000.0123.

4. J. Salat-Baroux, "Les avortements spontanés à répétition" [Recurrent Spontaneous Abortions], *Reproduction, Nutrition, Development* 28, no. 6B (1988): 1555–68, https://rnd.edpsciences.org/articles/rnd/abs /1988/10/RND_0181-1916_1988_28_6B_ART0002/RND_0181 -1916_1988_28_6B_ART0002.html; "5 Things You Should Know about Recurrent Miscarriages," *USC Fertility* (blog), https://uscfertility .org/5-things-know-recurrent-miscarriages.

5. Togas Tulandi, "Patient Education: Miscarriage (Beyond the Basics), *UpToDate*, last updated June 1, 2021, https://www.uptodate.com /contents/miscarriage-beyond-the-basics?search=miscarriage%20 beyond%20the%20basics&source=search_result&selectedTitle=1~150 &usage_type=default&display_rank=1#H1.

6. Johnna Nynas et al., "Depression and Anxiety Following Early Pregnancy Loss: Recommendations for Primary Care Providers," *Primary Care Companion for CNS Disorders* 17, no. 1 (January 2015), doi:10.4088/ PCC.14r01721.

7. E. W. Freeman, A. S. Boxer, K. Rickels, R. Tureck, and L. Mastroianni, "Psychological Evaluation and Support in a Program of In Vitro Fertilization and Embryo Transfer," *Fertility and Sterility* 43, no. 1 (1985): 48–53, doi: 10.1016/s0015-0282(16)48316-0.

Appendix A: CDC Screening Recommendations and Considerations for STDs

1. "Screening Recommendations and Considerations," Centers for Disease
    Control and Prevention, last reviewed June 6, 2022, https://www.cdc
    .gov/std/treatment-guidelines/screening-recommendations.htm.

Appendix B: Summary Chart of U.S.
Medical Eligibility Criteria for Contraceptive Use

1. "Summary Chart of U.S. Medical Eligibility Criteria for Contraceptive
    Use," Centers for Disease Control and Prevention, updated in 2020,
    https://www.cdc.gov/reproductivehealth/contraception/pdf/summary
    -chart-english-bw-508-tagged.pdf.

Index

Page numbers followed by *fig.* or *t.* refer to illustrations or tables, respectively.

About the Author

Nita Landry, MD, known as "Dr. Nita," is a board-certified obstetrician and gynecologist and a cohost of the Emmy Award–winning talk show *The Doctors*. She has also been featured as a go-to medical expert on television programs such as *Good Morning America* (with Strahan, Sara, and KeKe), the *Today* show, *Dr. Phil, Iyanla: Fix My Life*, and *CBS National News*.

After completing her medical residency, Dr. Nita became a traveling doctor, which took her to inner cities, rural towns, and Native American reservations from Alaska to New York, Minnesota to Texas, and lots of places in between. As she worked in clinics and hospitals across the country, she gained a wealth of knowledge and insight into the health issues most important to patient populations from all walks of life.

In addition to her work as a doctor, Dr. Nita enjoys inventing fun and innovative ways to deliver vital health information to the communities who need it, especially to those who are young, vulnerable, and underserved. As a frequent speaker on college campuses and at events across the country, she is committed to helping teens and young adults become healthier, happier versions of themselves.

Dr. Nita enjoys listening to live music, relaxing on the beach, and spending time with her friends and family. And she is a huge fan of New Orleans cuisine.

For more information, visit her website: drnitalandry.com.